NOTES OF GRATITUDE

———————

This book has been a loving creation inspired and produced by the help of countless beautiful souls in my life. There are several unnamed clients, family members, and friends that have supported me through this project and I am grateful to you all!

To the ones that have gone above and beyond:
Melodie—I am in awe of the depth of your heart and spirit. Thank you so much for reading my scribbles and encouraging me to move forward with this work. You are an inspiration to all who are blessed to be in your life.

Carrie, Kristi, and Candice—without your red pens I would be nowhere! I am deeply grateful for the time that you spent sculpting my words to convey my message in a meaningful manner. I value your opinions greatly, and I could never have done this without my creative collaboration team!

Kelly Webb Photography—thank you for the time and effort you contributed to make the graphics and pictures a reflection of the message of the book! www.kellyswebb.com

Thank you for your creative design and hours spent to make this book beautiful!
Hammdkhalid@gmail.com

DEDICATION

———————

This book is lovingly dedicated to Kent Bowen.
My dreams were only dreams until you challenged me to turn them into reality. You are by far the best teacher, coach, and mentor that has ever graced my life. I could never repay you for the confidence you have helped to instill in me. The direction of my career and success is a direct result of your presence in my life. Thank you!

REAL RESULTS FOR WOMEN WITH TYPE 2 DIABETES

—————

—————

978-0-692-97638-8)

Printed in the United States of America

Table of Contents

REAL RESULTS!

for Women with Type 2 Diabetes

by *Jessica Sutterfield*

ALL **ABOARD!**
Bikini Boot Camp **BEGONE!**

This book is not for the "Bikini Body" or the "Gym Rat" (although kudos to you ladies!).

This book is for the thousands of women wearing plus size clothing. For women being told by their doctors to lose weight ASAP, and get their Type 2 Diabetes under control.

For women who can't afford weight loss surgery, but can't afford to stay at their current weight. For women who have tried to lose weight and are scared to admit they don't think they can, but who really want to love their bodies again.

If you fall into any or all of those categories, welcome to the travel club! In this travel club, we are taking a 28-day health journey together. I am your personal Siri on this journey and I will lead you with my warrior ethos!

LEAVE NO 'WO'MAN BEHIND (Just leave half her '"behind" ' behind).

We are packing your bags (with clothes several sizes smaller) and bidding you *bon voyage* on your health journey to a vibrant, healthier, and more confident version of you (with better HGA1C results as well!).

We are going to be spending the next 28 days together on this journey. Have you ever noticed that when you travel with people, you end the trip with a clearer picture of who they are than when you began the trip? In my previous career as a teacher, I attended conferences in Austin, Texas, with all the third grade teachers in the school district. By the end of the four days, I would know their favorite beverages; their children's names, ages, and which sports they played; their husband's snoring habits; and their shoe sizes! We will have the same bonding experience on this journey together. I am going to let you in on my personal secrets, tips, and tricks to help you reach your health goals. And I can't wait to hear your success story!

During these next 28 days I will be your personal Siri! I have a roadmap to a Type 2 Diabetes-free destination, and I know how far it is to the next gas station. I know where all the awesome coffee shops are along the way, and where the detours and construction zones are. I have your personal roadmap to a destination without Type 2 Diabetes and your packing list is provided. All you have to do is check each item off the list and let the journey begin! Welcome aboard!

MEET YOUR **SIRI**
All About the **AUTHOR**

Who is this Jessica, and why should I listen to her?

"I don't want a Barbie doll telling me how to change my body."
-Melissa

I Am..............	I Have..............
A runner, a triathlete, and a crossfitter	HGA1C levels on the cusp of pre-diabetes
A certified Personal trainer with over a decade in the business	Trouble losing weight
Certified in metabolic efficiency and a graduate of the Institute of Integrative Nutrition	Over-exercised to lose weight
Partnered with local physicians to teach their patients how to exercise and eat	Been the chubby girl in school
Honored to have helped thousands of clients lose weight and keep it off	Tried diet pills and calorie restriction to see the number I wanted on the scale
On a health journey to a better version of me	Hypothyroidism and have had crazy sugar cravings
The owner of a thriving fitness and nutrition business	Had about 10 extra pounds that I'd like to lose
Learning to love my body as it is today	Struggled with self-image since elementary school

Greetings and Blessings! I am Jessica and I am not a Barbie Doll.
Every word in this roadmap is a tool that I use daily to keep myself on the path to health and wellness.

> ## *"Your Genetics load the gun. Your Lifestyle pulls the trigger."*
> ## *--Dr. Oz*

I am the embodiment of that infamous quote!

The "I Have" column is mostly due to the blood and bones I was given. The "I Am" column is a direct result of my daily conscious choices to keep that trigger locked, avoiding 50 extra pounds and Type 2 Diabetes. My gun is loaded for Type 2 Diabetes! You could say I am predestined to be overweight. But I am living proof the I Ams have as much influence as the I Haves.

I have been teased for being the "Snobby Eater," have been dubbed the "Healthy Hypochondriac," and of course, the "Health Nut." But I hold my head high and wear these nametags proudly. They are the only reason I am not 50 or 100 pounds overweight.

It is because of my daily decisions that I do not have autoimmune conditions, fibromyalgia, or similar conditions.

It is because of my adherence to the roadmap that I can swim, bike, run, deadlift, hike, play catch, and climb stairs.

My body is not perfect but it is healthy and functional. If you have any of my "Haves" above then you can join me on the I Am side. All you have to do is make the daily decision to stay on this road.

In Health, Love, and Hope,
Jessica

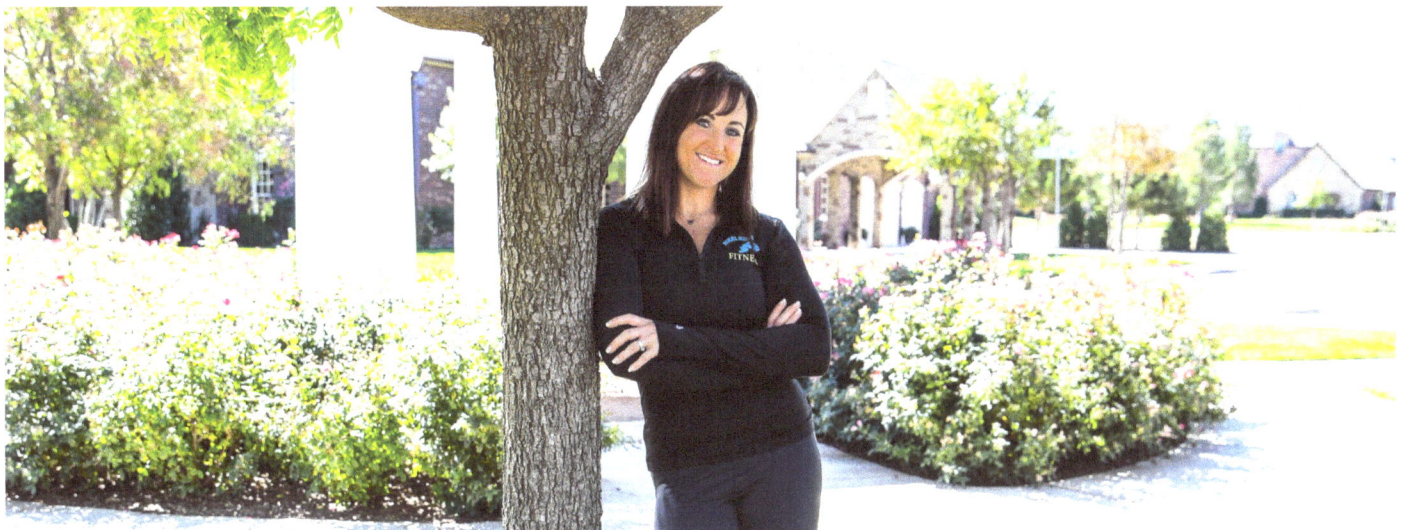

Chapter 1:

DESTINATION **VACATION**

Mirror Image of Your **Health Journey**

When you plan a destination vacation, you plan with the end in mind. You pack sandals and floppy hats for the beach in Maui and snow boots and beanies for the slopes in Breckenridge. For a vacation of a lifetime you begin fantasizing and visualizing the vacation for months or years in advance. The anticipation is often times more intense than the realization of the vacation.

A few years ago we took a family vacation to Belize. We started a year in advance by scheduling that week off from work. We booked our flight reservations, lodging, and made arrangements to board the family pets during our absence. Six months in advance we finalized the details of our trip by planning an excursion into the jungle, a tour of the Mayan ruins, and a day of ocean fishing. We had to start the passport process for our kids since that was their first international travel experience. We also did some Google researching to find the best places to eat and the prettiest places to lie on the beach. Three months from takeoff was time for some shopping! Now that we had an itinerary, we knew that each of us needed one or two pairs of sandals, walking shoes and hiking shoes, swimsuits for each day on the beach, a cute hat for the ocean excursion (for me), and long sleeves and jeans for mosquito protection on the jungle tour. As we landed in Belize, we realized an entire year of anticipation had arrived for this one moment. The magazine cover-worthy cabana sitting on miles of white sand with the turquoise waves lapping at the shore was worth every minute of that year-long wait! Yes, that destination was climactic! But we had spent 365 days planning for those ten short days. A scrapbook full of memories and pictures to last a lifetime was worth every minute of planning and every dollar spent, but we could not have gotten there without the journey.

Your health journey is a mirror of my journey to Belize. It takes intentional planning and follow through with attention to details and patience. But the stark difference between my vacation and your health journey on Earth is that there is no destination. There is only the journey. The destination is a mirage in the desert. I can't wiggle my nose like Samantha from Bewitched and give you a perfect body. But as your personal Siri, I can lead you on a journey to a body that you love, and a body that functions how you want it to function that can carry you through your adventures for the next thirty, forty, and fifty years of your life!

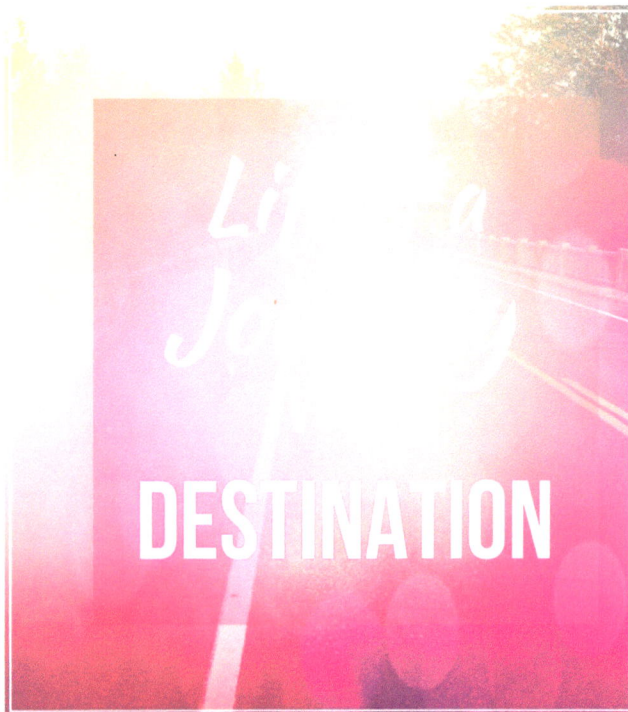

Chapter 2:

"THE JOURNEY, NOT THE DESTINATION, IS THE PRIZE." -JESSICA SUTTERFIELD

Learning to Value **the Journey**

I wished during the Belize prep time that I had an "Easy Button" to push. Keeping track of all the to-dos was exhausting! I recently took an eight-hour drive to visit a dear friend in Boulder, Colorado, and as I squirmed in my seat from my tight back and numb toes, I found myself yearning to punch an "Easy Button" to time warp me from Amarillo to Boulder. But it dawned on me that trying to speed up the trip was just speeding away minutes of my life.

The journey itself had value; I worked on this book the entire time. And when I quit being in such a hurry to arrive in Boulder, I took the time to look around at the beautiful scenery. Undulating hills, a herd of buffalo, picturesque creeks cutting through statuesque mountains; that journey had value, just as this 28-day journey has value to you. My eight-hour trip was a beautiful time for me to take in new scenery and spend some quiet time reflecting.

This 28-day journey is filled with healing movement and delicious food! If there was an easy button to time warp you beyond these 28-days I wouldn't even give it to you! Why?
Because this 28-day journey is what is valuable, not how you feel on day 28! In these 28-days you

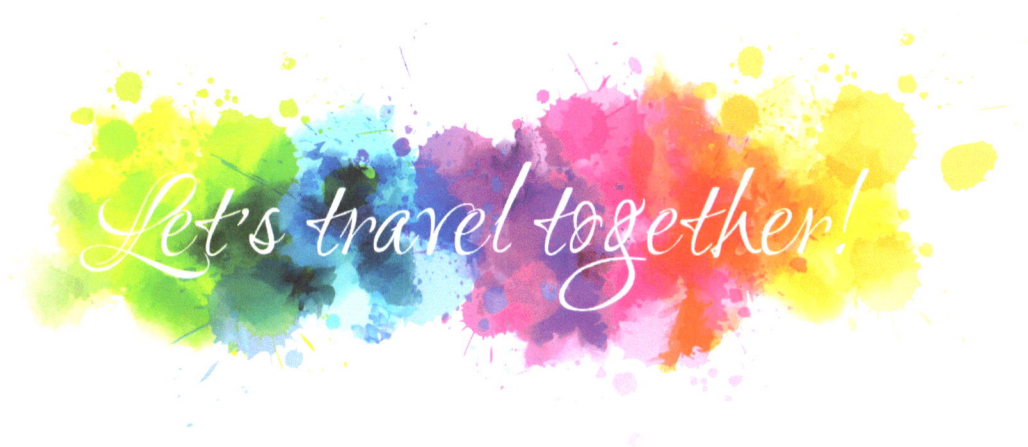

Let's travel together!

are going to realize that you can live the rest of your life eating, drinking, and moving like this! And you don't have to live with Type 2 Diabetes or fifty extra pounds anymore! You will recapture your body from this condition, so that the remainder of your journey (without me as your personal Siri) will be as beautiful, memorable and valuable as my eight-hour drive to Boulder.

Chances are you are reading this book because your journey is currently compromised due to the limitations of Type 2 Diabetes: excess weight, blood sugar crashes, lethargy, and a myriad of pills to take each morning. But you don't have time for these setbacks. You have kids or grandkids' soccer games to watch, retirement parties and baby showers to plan, benefit dinners to go to, trips across the country to take. You have places to go, and your body is going to have to get you there.

Your doctor tells you he will increase your medications if you do not lose some weight now—and you would if you knew how. It used to be easier when you were younger! But now there are diet pills, diet powders, and warning labels against said diet pills and powders. There are exercise classes, but you are uncomfortable in the gym and so much of it hurts your body right now. Each prescription you take comes with a litany of all the potential adverse side effects from taking the medication.

Don't let your dreams be only dreams!

You are tired of the gimmicks on TV and the supermodel fitness exercise videos on your social media feed. You are ready to get to your health destination, but you don't have plane tickets, you don't have the right clothes packed, and nothing in your house is in order. You can't start your health journey until you tie up your loose ends and prepare for your journey!

In these 28 days you will tie up those loose ends. You will lose weight, increase your stamina, get off some medications, and get your doctor off your back! You would not enjoy Maui if you had the flu. Similarly, you can't enjoy the life you are living if you have Type 2 Diabetes or fifty extra pounds.

Better things are Coming

THE ELLIE ENCOUNTER

Body Naming, Body Blaming, **Body Shaming**

I have been in the fitness industry for over a decade, and through my interactions with thousands of women, I am here to tell you that 99% of the female population are not only unsatisfied with their bodies, they despise their bodies! Women who are athletes, women who need to gain ten pounds, women who need to lose ten, fifty, over one hundred pounds have all sat in front of me and complained about something that they hate about their own body. I started to see a pattern in women (myself included) that I call Body Blaming, Body Naming, or Body Shaming. I want to share an inside view of what this Body Blaming, Naming and Shaming looks like in real life. This Ellie Encounter was my epiphany to understanding the minds of women and how they view their bodies, as well as being my impetus for creating this 28-day plan.

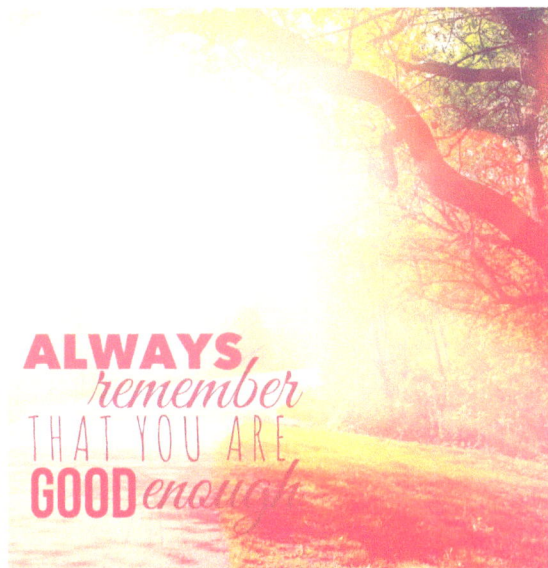

It was a typical Tuesday morning inside our local gym. People were hurrying in to sweat and hurrying out to work. The sun was shining through the windows and as the three gals I was training took their one-minute break in our Tabata set, we all noticed a woman outside on the sidewalk. And by "we noticed" I mean the four of us, the other three people walking down the sidewalk, and the half dozen men around the bench press stations. Everyone was hard pressed to not outright stare at the tan, twenty-something with bleached blonde hair sporting nothing but a sports bra and spandex booty shorts. She was 5'7" and had a better six pack than any I'd ever seen. Not only was she tall and lean, she embodied the term "ripped." This is not as common of a sight in Amarillo as it may be in other parts of the country, and the emotions her presence awakened in the ladies I was training and inside of me was eye opening.

When the woman continued standing outside instead of coming in, Sarah, an overweight mid-forties successful business professional piped up, "Maybe she's going to the doctor's office next door cause that's what I wear to appointments!"

Everyone snickered and Erica, a shy thirty-something stay-at-home mom, retorted, "Must be nice to be a twenty-year-old with no stretch marks and a thyroid that works!"

"Wow, her whole body is the size of my left thigh!" was the response from Tina, a very athletic business owner.

"Okay girls, that minute break turned into a three-minute break; back to work!" I teased as I directed them back to their kettlebells.

I cannot attest to what was going on inside any of their minds, only what was spoken. But I can tell you what was going on inside my mind. When I saw her, my heart sank to my knees and I felt the demon of self-deprecation land heavily on my shoulders. In the span of fifteen seconds, here are the thoughts that flew through my mind:

> *I wish I looked like that.*
> *I can't believe I let myself get this out of shape.*
> *I hope she doesn't come in here.*
> *She clearly knows more about exercise and nutrition than I do.*
> *I hope she doesn't come in here.*
> *Why am I even a trainer if I can't look like that?*
> *I hope she doesn't come in here.*
> *I'm so sick of how my legs look, I miss my muscles.*
> *I need to rerun my bloodwork and see if something is off with me.*
> *I hope she doesn't come in here.*

Now ladies, I'm sure many of you can relate to that torrential downpour of negative self-talk. But get this:

I can do pull-ups.
I win triathlons.
I can trail run, play basketball, and I don't look bad in a bikini.

At that moment when I heard my clients' comments while listening to that voice inside my head, it dawned on me: If I wanted to slither into a corner and hate her for her six pack—how did the other women in the gym feel? How do women feel every time they see social media posts from lean fitness celebrities doing burpees in sports bras while raving about the newest Bikini Bootcamp to join?

What body blaming scenarios flit through their minds? "It's not my fault, I've had four kids." Or, "Who cares if I eat donuts? My husband doesn't notice me anyway."

What body naming coping mechanisms emerge? "She looks like a stripper." "She's probably jacked up on diet pills." "She looks like a man with those biceps." "I'm sure she's bulimic."

What body shaming words do they use on themselves? "You are ugly, I can't believe you let yourself go." "You can't even wear shorts to the pool with that cellulite—forget about a swimsuit."

 What I realized is that as women our self-worth is inherently tied to our body image. Some women beat themselves up, some lash out against the women of whom they are envious, and some play the victim. Whatever the response is, the internal mechanism is the same.

I WANT TO FEEL BETTER IN MY BODY.

This encounter opened my eyes to the realization that we are each on our own Health Journey. There are women who need help to change their bodies, and I know how to help them. I have the roadmap to get them there.

A Flower
does not think of
competing
with the flower
next to it.
It just blooms.

THE ROADMAP

Theory of the **Scale**
Measurement **How-To**

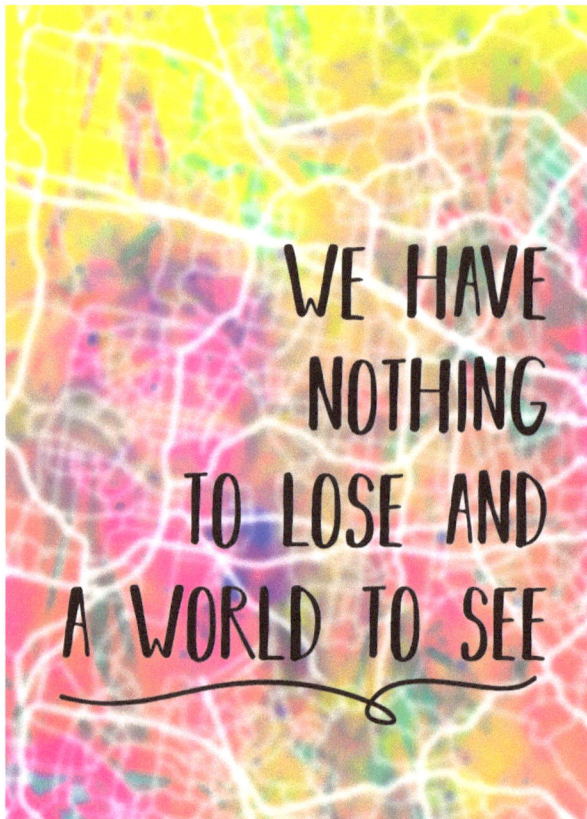

Now that you understand how this roadmap came to existence, it's time to get you packed up and on the road to a healthier version of you! Here is the to-do list for today:

1) *Take before pictures*
2) *Take before measurements*
3) *Get your starting weight*

For those of you who just rolled your eyes and decided to skip this chapter,

I am talking to you!

WE HAVE NOTHING TO LOSE AND A WORLD TO SEE

Yes, seeing the pictures can make you feel vulnerable. Getting your weight and measurements can cause anxiety to rise, but for the love of butter,

DO NOT SKIP THIS PIECE!

There is sunlight through this tunnel, I promise! And you will never regret seeing your progress. A detailed description and pictures of how to take the starting data are included at the end of this chapter. For now, humor me and read my theory of the scale. By the time you are done with this next section, all of your excuses and reasons for why you don't want to get your starting data will have vanished.

Theory of the scale

Whether you have 50 or 100 pounds to lose, it can seem daunting if you only look at the number on the scale. The number on the scale does have value but only as it relates to the changes in your body composition, specifically the changes in your lean mass and your fat mass. I do want you to weigh on Days 1, 14, and 28, but please refrain from weighing every day as fluctuations can be alarming and discouraging. The truest picture will be comparing Day 1 to Day 28.

The measurements you take will provide a clearer picture of your overall change and success. Many vitamin companies and gyms have free body composition scales which can be a great tool.

The important thing with recording weight is to use the same scale.

Either weigh at home and do your own measurements both times, or go to the same vitamin store and use the same machine both times. Do not use the scale in your doctor's office and then your home scale or vice versa. This will give you mixed data, and a scale that has not been calibrated is synonymous to throwing a bunch of nails on a highway and waiting for the tires to blow. It is also important to weigh and measure at the same time of the day and in the same clothing.

Contrary to misinterpretations, fat does not "turn into muscle." The principle that this misleading concept is trying to get across is that as lean muscle mass increases, the fat mass decreases. By following the 28-day movement and eating plan, you will preserve and even gain lean muscle and bone density as your body will be burning and eliminating fat.

As you build your lean muscle mass and bone density with the workouts in the 28-day plan, you create a more efficient metabolic system. Simply put, you are laying pavement on an old caliche country road.   As your body metabolizes the clean foods in the 28-day plan, you "unclog" your internal roadway system. Inflammation decreases, stress hormones balance, and you are soon on a smooth interstate highway with no potholes and no construction cones. The weight loss comes from the elimination of inflammation and the increase in metabolic efficiency. We're giving your body an oil change and putting on some new wheels!

If you choose to use a body composition test (which I highly recommend), the most important number is the body fat percent. The weight on the scale is akin to the dollar bill in China. It's meaningless without the currency exchange rate, and your exchange rate is the body fat percentage. The body fat percent compares the pounds of your body in muscle, bones, and water and compares it to the pounds of fat in your body. There are oodles of ideal body fat percent charts online. But I want you to understand that there is not a distinct number you are striving for during these 28 days. Instead, you are striving for 5-10% less body fat on day 28 than you had on day 1. That is progress in action! Remember, the destination is not the goal here: we are on the journey. Forward progress is progress. Our goal is to take steps toward the destination each day and avoid any "Rerouting, please make a U-turn as soon as possible!" mishaps.

Take Starting Measurements and Weight: Take measurements and weight on days 1, 14, and 28. Remember to always take these measurements first thing in the morning after you use the bathroom, but before you eat.

Take Before Pictures: Take your progress pictures first thing in the morning on days 1, 14, and 28 (just like your measurements and weight). Use these tips to get accurate comparison photos:

Find a place in your home with good natural light to take your pictures.

- *Wear the same thing—exactly—in all three pictures.*
- *Use the same lighting for all three sets of pictures.*
- *Stand the same distance from the camera in all three sets of pictures.*
- *Have your full body fill the frame of the photo. In other words, don't be too far away from the camera or you won't see your progress.*
- *Wear a sports bra and shorts if you're comfortable with that. The more of your body you can see, the more progress you'll see.*

HOW TO TAKE PERFECT MEASUREMENTS

Chest: Circumference of rib cage/chest at the nipple line

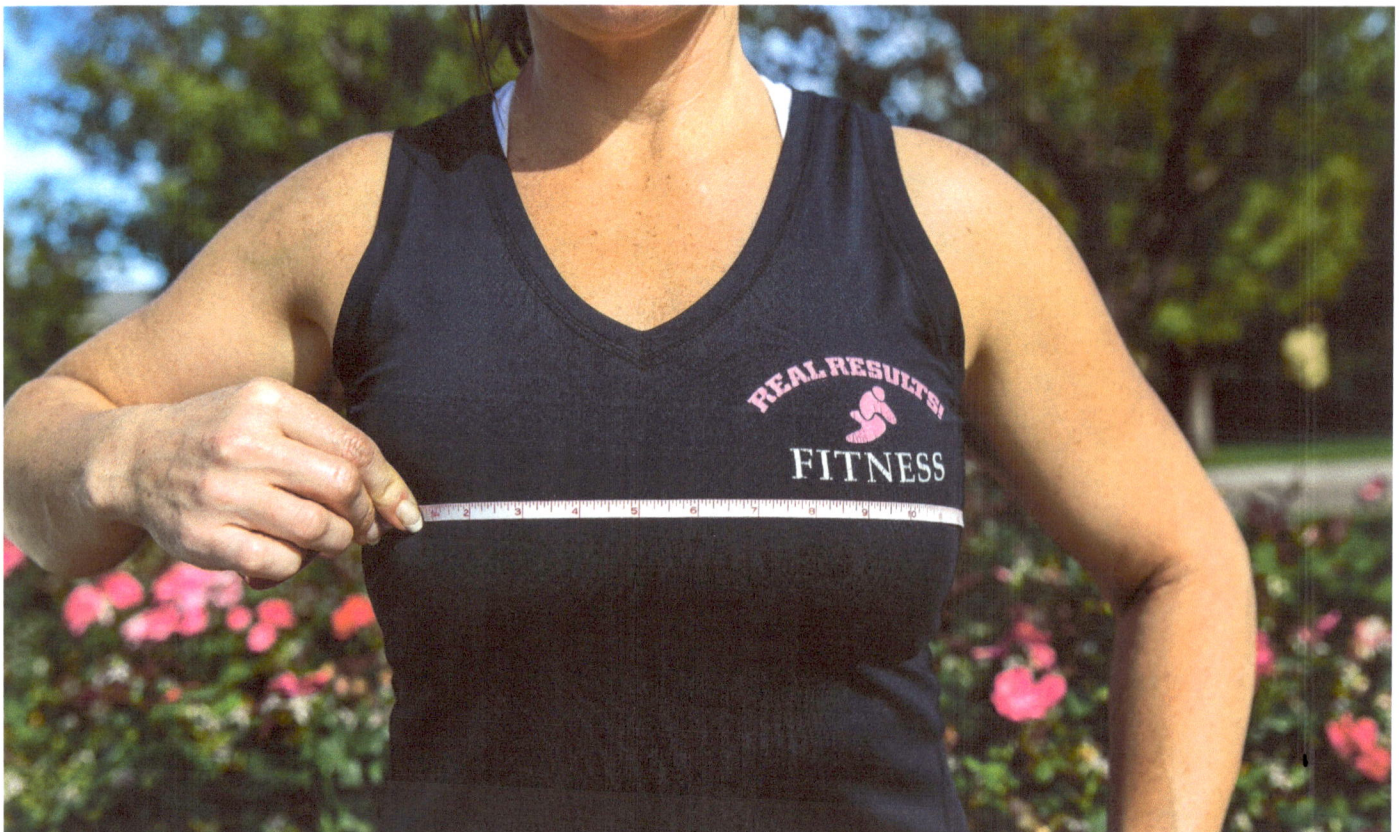

Waist: Circumference of waist at the smallest point—usually an inch or two below ribs

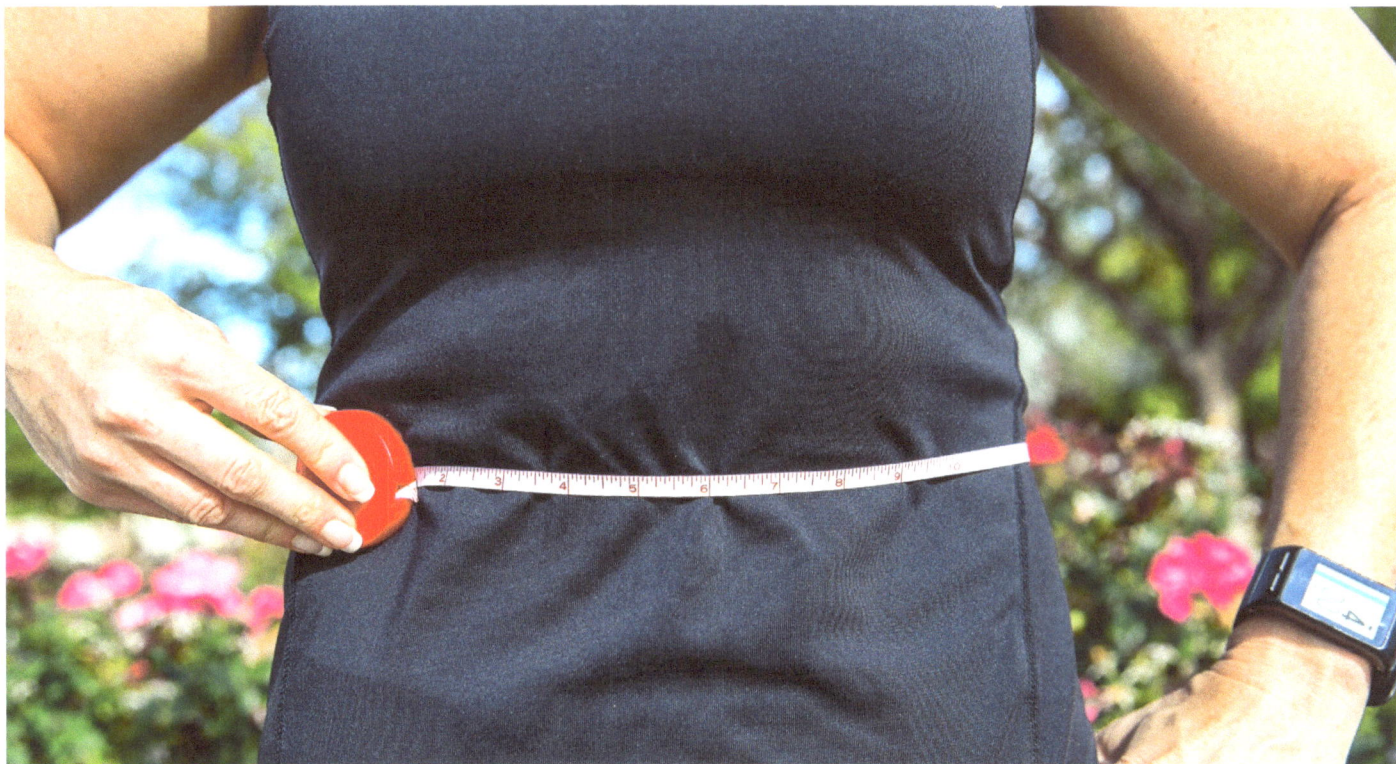

Belly Button: Circumference of stomach at the point that is level with belly button

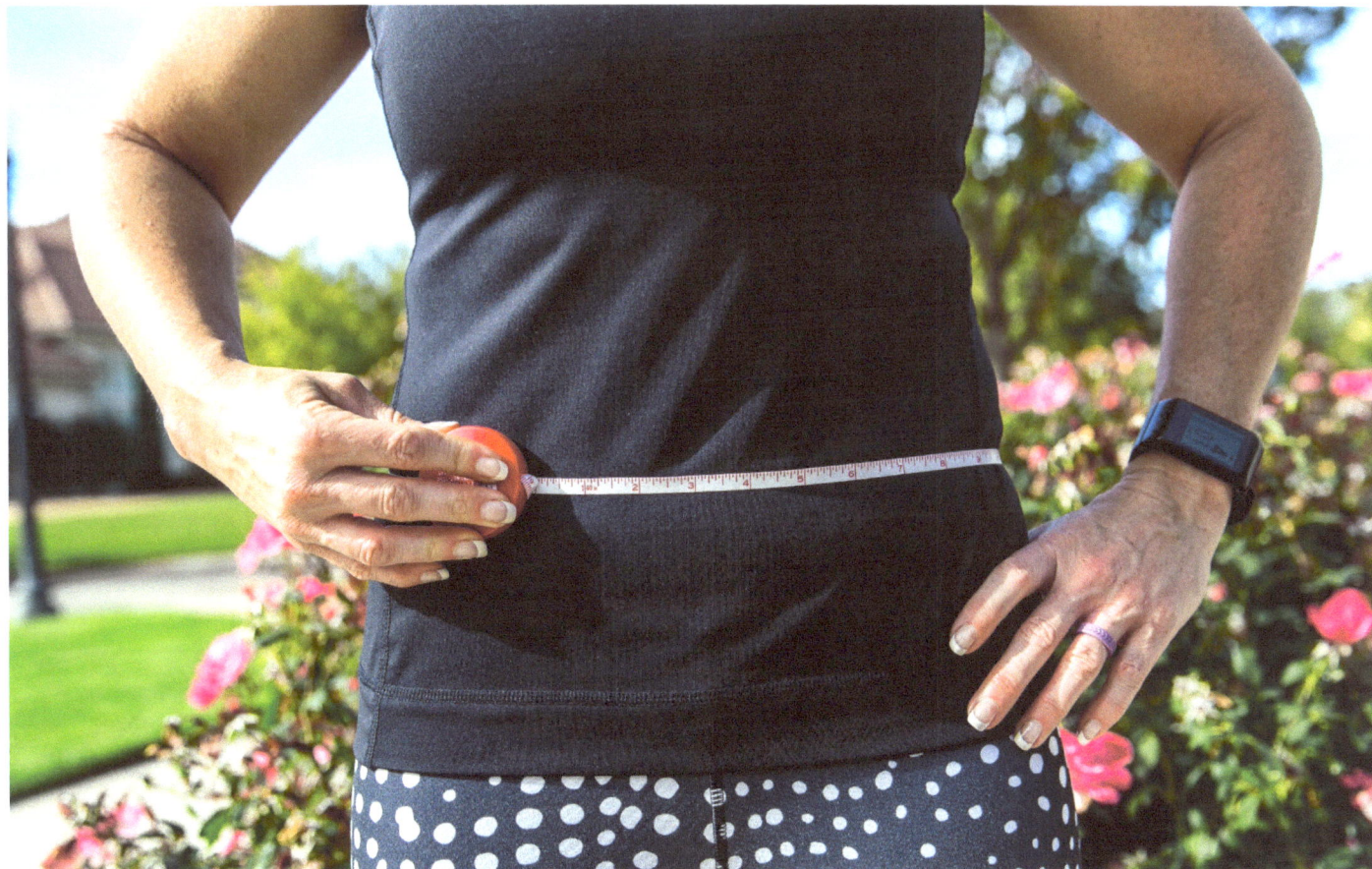

Glutes: Circumference of glutes/hips around the fullest part of glutes

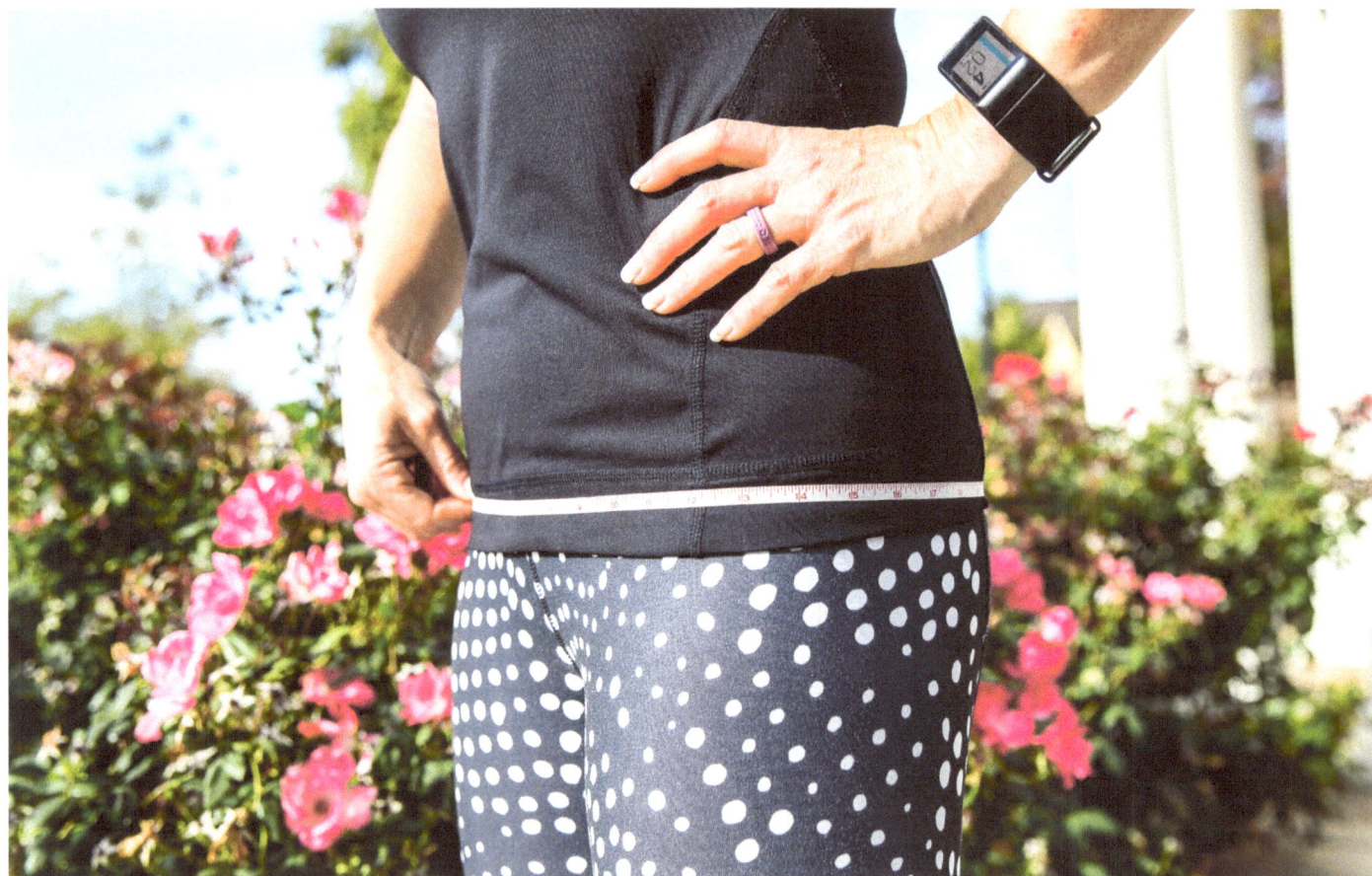

Right Thigh: Circumference of thigh around the fullest part

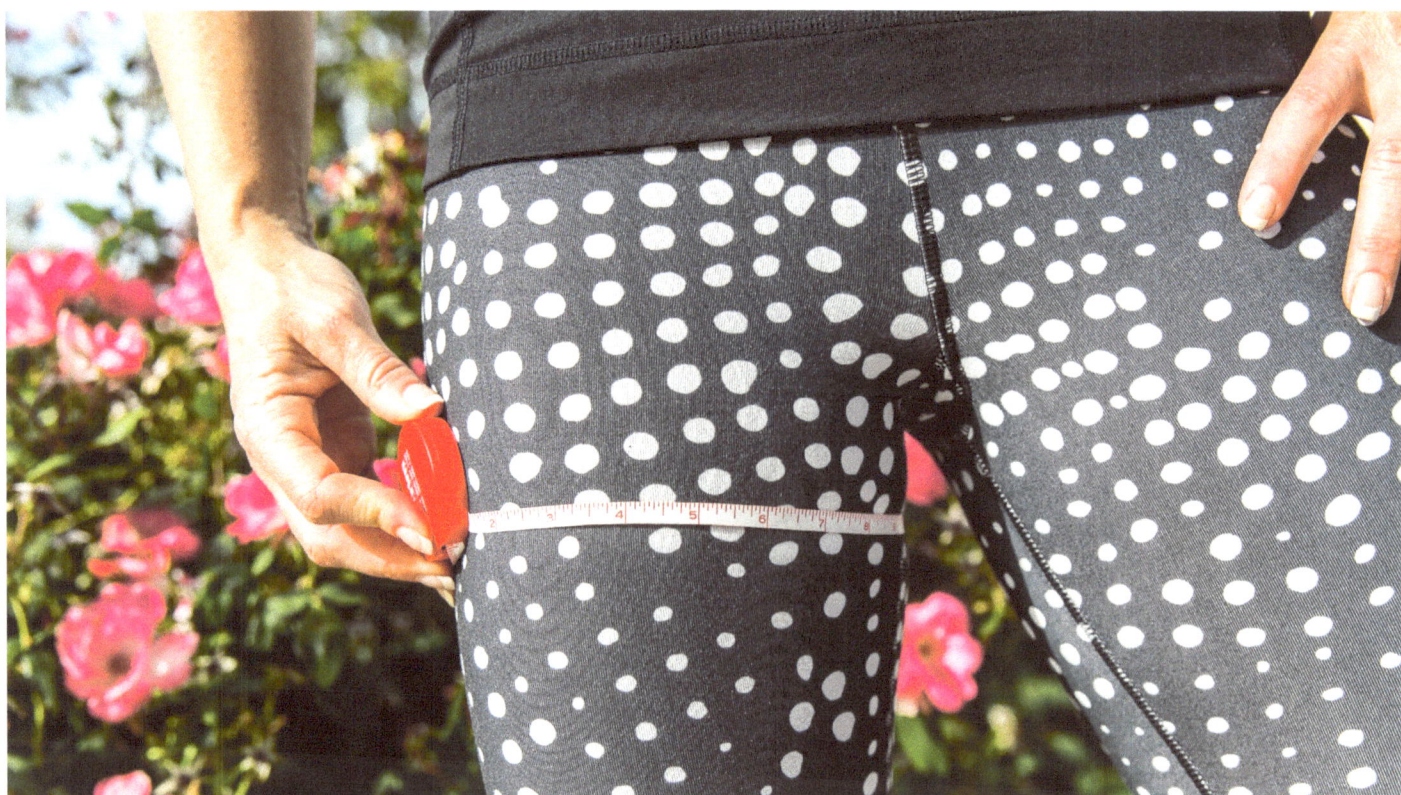

Right Calf: Circumference of calf around the fullest part

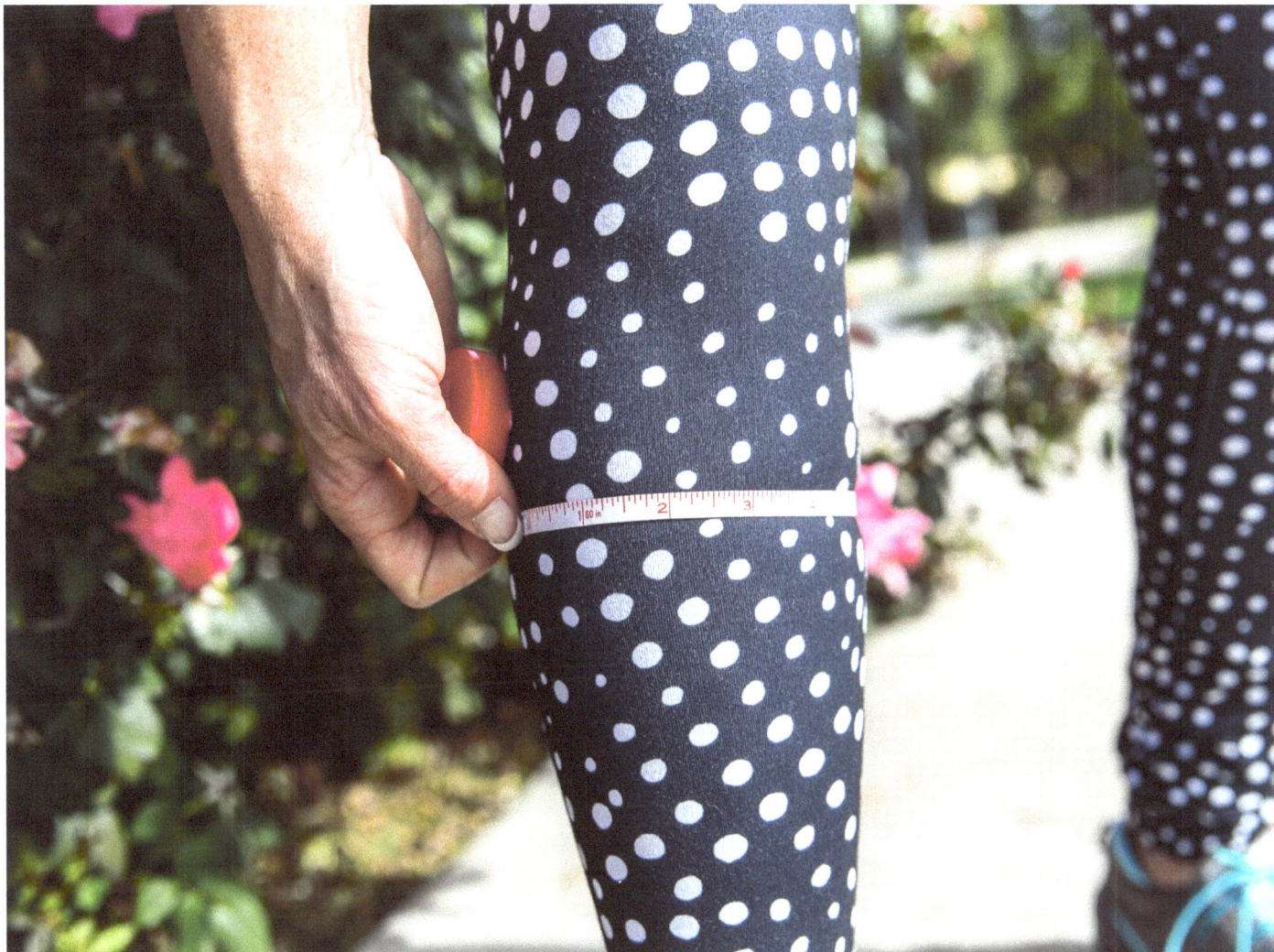

Right Arm: Circumference of arm half way between shoulder and elbow

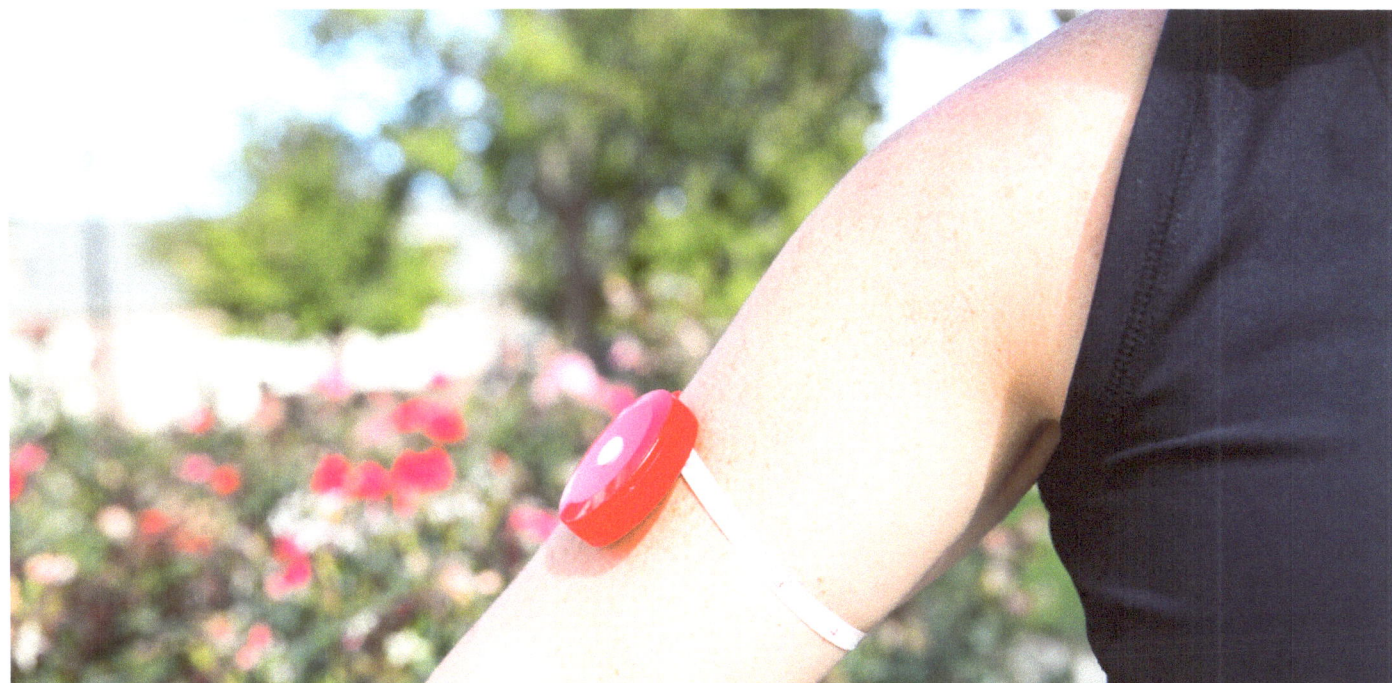

For all you eye rollers out there, now that you understand "why" we are taking starting data and you have the explanation of "how" to take them, get up and go do it! You will thank me in a few short days.

Chapter 5:

THE FATTENING FIVE

Thou Shalt Not List

I despise DON'T lists. Instead of veering me away, they beckon me like a bucket list!

Joshua Rosenthal, author of *Integrative Nutrition: Feed Your Hunger for Health and Happiness,* coined the term Bio-Individuality to encompass the philosophy of "there's no one-size-fits-all diet." Each person is a unique individual with highly individualized nutritional requirements. When it comes to food, although we may each gravitate towards different eating styles, *all* of us are better served by avoiding a cocktail of what I have named The Fattening Five.

ACESULFAME POTASSIUM

What is It?

Although innocent sounding enough, this laboratory creation is not a vitamin! It is a calorie-free sugar substitute measured at *two hundred times sweeter than sugar!*

Why don't I want it?

Realizing that consumers have become savvy to avoiding products with sugar, food companies now replace sugar with artificial sweeteners. All artificial sweeteners are distasteful—pun intended! But acesulfame potassium is in over 4,000 products and increasing daily so it is a major player that needs to be spotlighted as a "Thou Shalt Not."

Think about that birthday cake protein powder with 20 grams of protein and zero grams of sugar. Does it taste sweet? How can anything with zero grams of sugar taste sweet? Artificial sweeteners!

This super sweet creation has been shown in recent studies to increase body weight and alter the gut microbiome.

Where does it hide?

Protein powders and supplements
Diet drinks
Diet or Lite foods

SOYBEAN OIL

What is It?

Most people visualize lean vegetarians when they hear the word soy. Soybean oil is the polar opposite of that image. Soybean oil is a cheaply produced, highly processed, highly inflammatory omega-6 oil that houses dangerous trans fats.

Why don't I want it?

Food companies now reduce the serving size on the label since they know consumers have begun to avoid products with trans fats . Half a gram of trans fat per serving can still legally be marketed as trans-fat free. The trick is to see if the serving size is something tiny, like one cookie.

Recent studies called soybean oil out as being more obesogenic and diabetogenic than fructose! In the study published by the U.S. National Library of Medicine, soybean oil caused significant increases in weight gain, fat stores, diabetes, glucose intolerance, and insulin resistance, as well as contributing to fatty liver.

Where does it hide?

Vegetable oil
Lecithin (an emulsifier in many chocolates and candies)
Mayonnaise and salad dressings
Margarine
Non-Dairy coffee creamers
Cooking oils in many restaurants
Sauces
Boxed foods

SUCRALOSE

What is It?

Sucralose, commonly known as Splenda, is a laboratory-produced sweetener with a chemical structure more similar to DDT(pesticide) than sugar!

Why don't I want it?

Just like Ace K, the nickname for acesulfame potassium, sucralose is one of the most commonly used artificial sweeteners. If you can just remember to knock out acesulfame potassium and sucralose you will be reducing your artificial sweetener intake by leaps and bounds. Apples don't have ingredient labels, and whole foods won't have artificial sweeteners.

This super sweet creation has been shown in recent studies to stimulate appetite, increase carbohydrate cravings, and stimulate fat storage and weight gain.

Where does it hide?

Protein powders and supplements
Commercial baked goods
Non-alcoholic beverages
Chewing gum
Frozen dairy desserts
Fruit juices

MONOSODIUM GLUTAMATE (MSG)

What is It?

Sodium is natural and glutamate is naturally found in the body, therefore you might assume that Monosodium Glutamate must be healthy. This false conclusion is adding inches to your waistline daily! MSG is a chemically created flavor enhancer that is present in more than just Chinese food. Scarily and sadly, it is in most packaged products, sometimes under a pseudonym. (See chart below)

Why don't I want it?

Food companies make money when we make purchases. The best way to encourage us to make purchases is to make it irresistible. I could chow down on a party-sized bag of caramel-filled chocolate candies. But I could not chow down on the same volume of broccoli. This horrific concoction tricks your brain into thinking it is still hungry—the "stop eating" message never gets to your tongue—or your fork! Do people binge on cookie dough or carrots? There is a reason for this frantic "give me more" sensation, and it's a direct result of the *anti-appetite suppressant* addictiveness of MSG.

MSG makes you fat. It's been proven. "MSG consumption was positively, longitudinally associated with overweight development among apparently healthy Chinese adults." This study by the American Journal of Clinical Nutrition concurs with the sentiment from the Public Library of Science study, "The amount of dietary monosodium glutamate (MSG) is increasing worldwide, in parallel with the epidemics of metabolic syndrome. Parenteral administration of MSG to rodents induces obesity, hyperglycemia, hyperlipidemia, insulin resistance, and Type 2 Diabetes." Say good-bye to MSG today!

Where does it hide?

Seasoning packets
Sauces, marinades, dressings
"Natural" flavors
Beef, chicken, pork flavoring or bouillon
Maltodextrin
Carrageenan
Pseudonyms for MSG:
These ingredients here are just refurbished names of MSG.

Autolyzed Yeast	Calcium Caseinate	Gelatin
Glutamate	Glutamic Acid	Hydrolyzed Protein
Monopotassium Glutamate	Monosodium Glutamate	Sodium Caseinate
Textured Protein	Yeast Extract	Yeast Food
Yeast Nutrient		

MALTODEXTRIN

What is It?

Maltodextrin is carbohydrate starch processed from corn, wheat, rice, and potatoes. Most of the time it is sourced from corn and is used as a "filler" to give processed food more volume and fluff.

Why don't I want it?

The glycemic index measures how a carbohydrate-containing food raises blood glucose. Foods are ranked based on how they compare to glucose which sits at 100. Table sugar has a GI of 65 and maltodextrin's GI trumps both, weighing in at 110! The high GI of maltodextrin causes blood sugar to spike, and then our bodies store that excess glucose as fat.

This food additive has zero nutritional benefits. And it is generally combined with ingredients like brown rice syrup, high fructose syrup, wheat and oats, which you will learn on Day 27 is a recipe for turning your body into a fat-making machine!

Where does it hide?

Protein bars and powders
Cereals, cereal bars
Granola bars, snack bars
Commercial baked goods
Sauces
Processed foods like cookies, chips, pastries

There is one super simple way to know you are avoiding the Fattening Five, and that's by eating whole foods that don't come in boxes. When you are picking out cooking staples like seasonings, sauces, or protein powders (discussed in the next chapter!) be a label detective and make sure that you are choosing a clean product free from the Fattening Five. Definitely when you are at a restaurant, ask the wait staff which dishes are MSG-free before ordering.

SUPPLEMENTS

Nutrition or **Nonsense**

> *"Buy this powder to lose weight!"*
> *"These protein bars are the best for weight loss!"*

How many advertising campaigns do you see for raspberries? Or for avocados?

Whole foods don't get media attention or billboards. We are being told by the marketing industry that we need to buy powders and pills, but in most situations, if we eat whole foods our bodies can take care of themselves efficiently.

If your physician recommends a product after reviewing your lab results, then pay attention. But if you see a commercial or social media post touting the awesomeness of a "new and improved" supplement for weight loss think twice before purchasing. Have you been eating your daily greens? Have you been drinking half your body weight in ounces of water?

Spinach in powder form is always second to spinach on a fork.

Patch up any nutritional holes before looking for miracle products.

That said, I am frequently asked about supplemental products and my answer is almost always the same,

"Supplement don't Supplant."

Do I use a protein powder? **Yes, I do.**
Daily? **Nope.**
And more than once a day? **Never!**

Variety is the key to getting a balanced approach of micronutrients. Broccoli has a wonderful nutritional profile, but if we eat only broccoli then we are missing out on the micronutrients found in veggies like bell peppers, arugula, and green beans. The answer to the supplement question is to eat a variety of fruits, veggies, and proteins, and then use supplements when necessary.

Generally speaking, most of us can benefit from taking Probiotics, Digestive Enzymes, Vitamin D3, and Fish Oil. I am not saying that these products are necessary for you to make progress on your health journey, but as you are patching up the nutritional holes with our Nourishing Meal Map, these products have the potential to speed you along your way. Keep in mind that boycotting fast food will always make a bigger impact on your body than popping pills.

My only plea when you purchase protein powders and supplements is that you scan the ingredient label to be sure they are free from the Fattening Five. If your jug of creamy cookies and cream powder tastes "Oh So Sweet," but has zero grams of sugar, that is a red flag to be on the lookout for culprits like acesulfame potassium, sucralose, and other artificial flavors.

You can go to my website, http://realresultsfitness.net/index.php?page=book, for Amazon links to products that I have found to be free from the Fattening Five. There are other clean products on the market, you just have to be an ingredient detective!

Supplement	Why Would I Want It?	When Would I NOT Want it?
Probiotics	Probiotics are friendly microorganisms inhabiting our digestive tract that aid digestion through complex symbiosis between the gut, the bacteria, and the rest of our body. Potential health benefits include keeping our bowels regular, treatment of diarrhea, reduction of lactose intolerance, improved immune system, lower chances of colon cancer, and reduction of blood pressure and cholesterol.	Probiotics may result in mild flatulence, which should subside with continued use. They may be contraindicated for use with immunosuppressant medications.
Digestive Enzymes with Hydrochloric Acid (HCL)	Hydrochloric acid is the stomach acid that helps break down food and	Large amounts of hydrochloric acid may cause stomach irritation.

maintains the acidic environment in the digestive system necessary to kill "bad" bacteria, parasites, and pathogens that may be ingested with food.

Important for stimulating the pancreas and intestines to produce the bile and enzymes necessary to break down foods.

DIGESTIVE ENZYMES: Potential health benefits include supporting enhanced protein, carbohydrate, fat, fiber and dairy digestion, and promoting optimal nutrient bioavailability and absorption.

May be contraindicated for those with a history of peptic ulcers, gastritis, or gastrointestinal symptoms.

People taking nonsteroidal anti-inflammatory drugs (NSAIDs), cortisone-like drugs, or other medications that might cause a peptic ulcer should not take hydrochloric acid.

| Vitamin D3 | Vitamin D is available in a few foods and from sunlight exposure. It is an important factor in making sure your muscles, heart, lungs, and brain work well and that your body can fight infection. | Large doses of vitamin D can cause hypercalcemia. Signs include headache, weakness, nausea, vomiting, and constipation. Those with hyperparathyroidism or kidney disease are at particular risk. |

Potential health benefits include enhancing calcium absorption and retention, and supporting cardiovascular, colon, and cellular health.

Fish Oil-EPA/ DHA	**EPA AND DHA FROM FISH OIL:** Encourage cardiovascular health by supporting triglyceride and lipid metabolism, maintaining healthy blood flow, and promoting healthy platelet function Potential health benefits include balancing levels of inflammation in the body, and supporting joint function.	May cause burping, gastrointestinal upset or indigestion, nausea, diarrhea, or abdominal bloating. It has a mild blood thinning effect and may influence glucose metabolism in some individuals, typically at larger levels.

These supplements are all available without a prescription, and have dosage amounts on the bottles. Keep in mind, however, that the beautiful part of having a physician look at lab results to make supplement decisions is the confidence of knowing you aren't throwing money away on a pill that your body doesn't need!

For a list of functional medicine doctors near you, check out https://www.ifm.org/find-a-practitioner/

I also have a list of practitioners that I work with listed on my website at: www.RealResultsFitness.nethttp://realresultsfitness.net/index.php?page=book

Chapter 7:

INSTRUCTION MANUAL FOR **DAYS 1-28**

Each day has a Lifestyle Lesson or teaching point, your daily workout, and the meals for that day.

Use this as a daily 5-minute focus.

You don't have to read all 28-days at once, just the page that corresponds to your day.

For your convenience, all exercises, the full meal plan, and the weekly shopping lists are provided in the appendix section of the book.

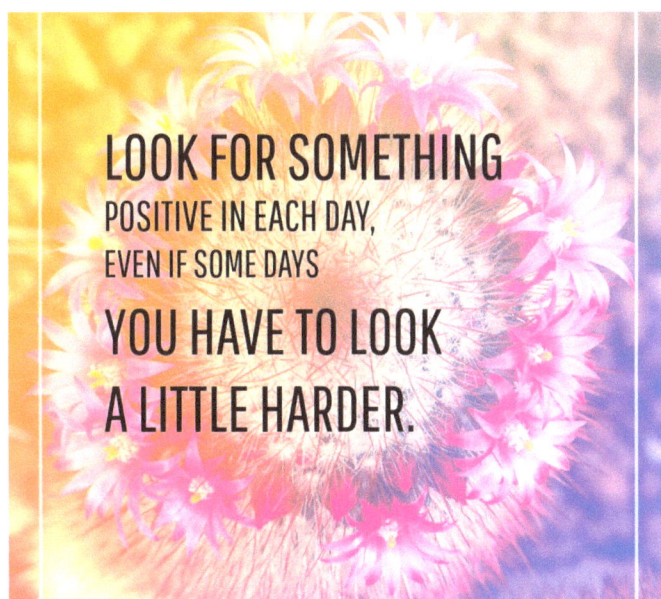

LOOK FOR SOMETHING POSITIVE IN EACH DAY, EVEN IF SOME DAYS YOU HAVE TO LOOK A LITTLE HARDER.

Day 1 Lifestyle Lesson:
To Thine Own Self Be True

Listen to your Inner Siri

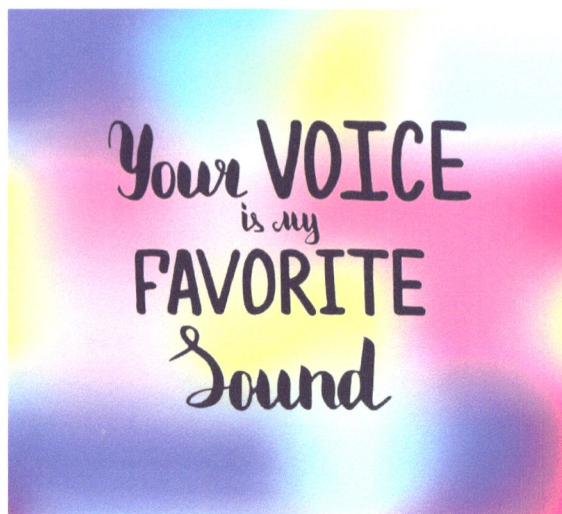

The first item on your packing list is to tune in to your Inner Siri. We each have a built-in navigation system. You can call it your guiding voice, intuition, or gut instinct. Regardless of what you call it, your Inner Siri, if you allow her, will lead you straight.

How does that translate to real life?

If you are following the meal plan and you start to notice that you feel bloated after your protein shake, tune into that; don't ignore it! Maybe your protein powder has a shellfish base for glucosamine in it, and your body isn't tolerating the shellfish influence. Or maybe your almond milk has carrageenan and it's irritating your digestive tract. To be the best you, you have to listen to you first and foremost. Your body does not have a voice so it speaks to you through physical means. Honor your body and she will honor you.

Day 1 Meals: **Refer to Chapter 10**

Day 1 Movement: 20-minute Strength Training
Refer to Chapter 9

Day 2 Lifestyle Lesson:
Don't Put Beer in the Fridge of an Alcoholic

Sugar and processed carbohydrates are every bit as addictive as narcotics and alcohol! Who in their right mind would put a six pack in the fridge of a friend coming home from rehab? This common sense applies to your pantry and your personal addictions as well. You know what sets you on a binge. Ruffles? Oreos? Whatever your vice is, remove it from your sight! Right now. I seriously mean right this instant. Get up, go to your fridge or pantry, and throw it away! The $2.50 you spent is not worth the hours and days of remorse you will feel.

Food for thought—Alcohol also triggers binge eating in many people. If you realize that a glass of wine or a beer causes you to fall face first into the bag of chips, then it is in your best interest not to partake. The empty calories and sugar present in alcoholic beverages are potholes on your highway. Avoid the potholes.

Day 2 Meals: **Refer to Chapter 10**

Day 2 Movement: 10 Minute H.I.I.T. Training
Refer to Chapter 9

You are inspiring beautiful courageous amazing

Day 3 Lifestyle Lesson:
Fix the Flat Tire

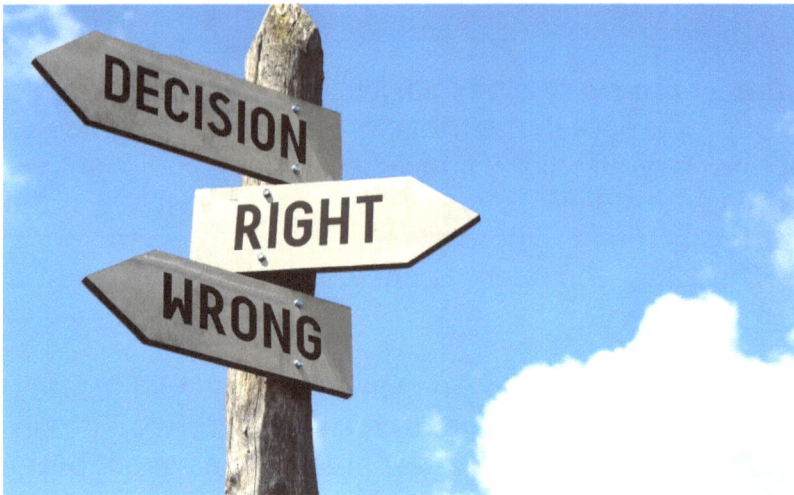

"Ugh! I don't have time for a flat!"

We have all been there. How do you respond?

You walk around to the back tire, and after seeing that it's flat, you pull out your Swiss Army knife and slash the other three tires.

"There! That tire is trashed, so I might as well trash the other three!"

Not likely!

If you have a flat tire you might kick it, complain loudly, and call to have it fixed. You are annoyed and late, but you are not stupid. "I ate the donut in the break room this morning. I am so mad at myself. Ugh!! I cannot believe I already messed up. I might as well have the peach cobbler at lunch. A vanilla Coke? Sure. Why not? This day is trashed already. I think I'll just have Taco Villa tonight since I blew the day anyway." This stupidity in thinking leads to more weight gain and self-deprecation than anything I have ever witnessed. The donut was 500 calories of junk. The donut, cobbler, soda, and fast food comes to a whopping 2,300 calories of junk, shame, and sabotage! You can stop with the bill for one flat tire or you can have the bill for four flat tires. Ladies, make the smart decision.

Day 3 Meals: **Refer to Chapter 10**

Day 3 Movement: Gossip Walk **Refer to Chapter 9**

Day 4 Lifestyle Lesson:
You are Not a Garbage Disposal

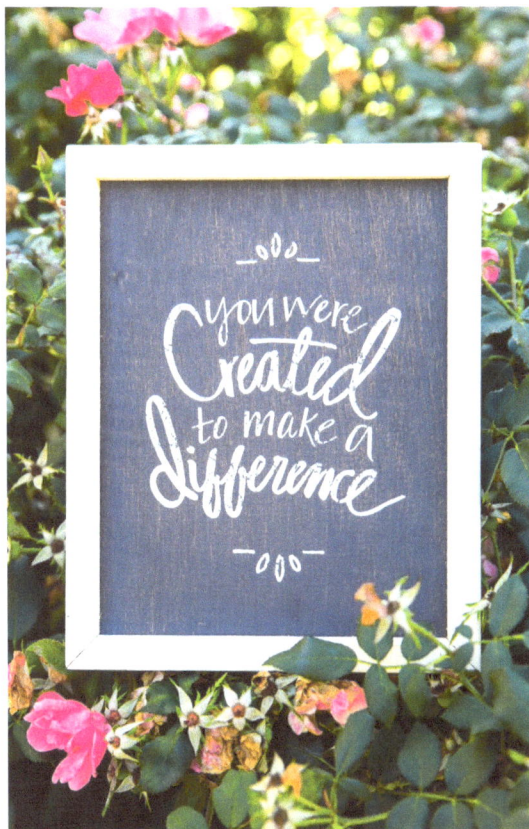

Last night's Spicy Salmon was sooooo mouthwateringly good! You enjoyed every bite! When you began the dish clearing process you ate the leftover piece of salmon off your daughter's plate. "I don't want to waste that expensive fish!" And the two pieces stuck on the skillet. "It has to be a sin to throw this away." And the avocado slice left in the salad bowl. "It'll be brown in the morning." In your post meal clean up you just added another 250 calories to your already full and satisfied tummy! Sound familiar? Stop and make a U-turn! This is the WRONG WAY. There are DO NOT ENTER signs all over this road! You are not a garbage disposal. Your stomach is not a trash can. You are a work in progress. When you are finished eating a meal and there are two big bites of leftover filet or chocolate cake on the plate, I see that you have three options:

1) Eat it even though you are full so it doesn't go to waste (a.k.a. garbage disposal)
2) Wrap it up and save the rest for tomorrow
3) Throw it in the trash can

If you cannot stomach the idea of trashing food, then for the love of butter, put it in Tupperware and save it! But do not relegate your body to the duty of trash can or garbage disposal. That food will come out of you into the toilet or go into a landfill, but either way it is refuse on the way out. Do not be a garbage disposal.

Day 4 Meals: **Refer to Chapter 10**

Day 4 Movement: 20-minute Strength Training
Refer to Chapter 9

Day 5 Lifestyle Lesson:
Tomorrow is a Redo

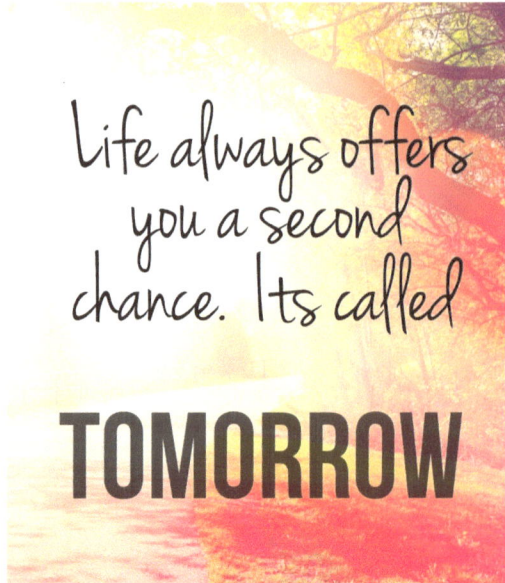

Life always offers you a second chance. Its called TOMORROW

Remember that easy button I vowed never to give you? Well, I have something better for you! It is a reset button and you have one every morning! You are going to have weddings, BBQs, and holidays. Embrace these occasional situations as a joyful sliver of your life. Have a piece (not 3) of wedding cake, enjoy a sausage at the company BBQ, and do not skip out on your favorite holiday treat. The trick to living life in balance is simply that: balance. Have that treat and then push the reset button in the morning. Eat clean all day long with a clear conscience knowing that you enjoyed the party last night and you are caring for your body all day today.

The reset button is a yellow blinking caution light. If you have cake every day your reset button wears out. Remember to focus on balance.

Day 5 Meals: **Refer to Chapter 10**

Day 5 Movement: **30 Minute Bubble Bath**

Day 6 Lifestyle Lesson:
Train Your Eyes to Train Your Brain

I think it is excessive and demeaning to weigh and measure your food every day (it evokes images to me of rationing lines in prisons or school cafeterias!). However, I do see relevance in spending two to three days measuring each serving to be sure your eyes are being truthful. Using your cruise control protects you from unintentionally busting over the speed limit. Overconsumption, even of healthful foods, will work against your goals of shrinking your waistline. To prevent those red and blue flashing lights in the rear-view mirror, use my 3-day map for retraining your eyes:

- For the next three days use a small salad plate instead of a large dinner plate. (Who decided the dinner plate should be the size of choice for serving meals anyway?)
- For the next three days use a measuring cup or measuring spoons for every meal, snack, veggie serving, dressing, and drink to recalibrate your eyes. We have a tendency to drastically underestimate the amount of food we scoop out of a serving dish.
- Start to eyeball portions with your hand. This graphic can help you make serving decisions at buffets, Sunday pot lucks, and even at home.
- Protein and starchy veggies = palm of hand
- Leafy veggies = entire outstretched hand fingertip to wrist
- Nuts/nut butters = closed fist

Day 6 Meals: Refer to Chapter 10

Day 6 Movement: 10 Minute H.I.I.T. Training
Refer to Chapter 9

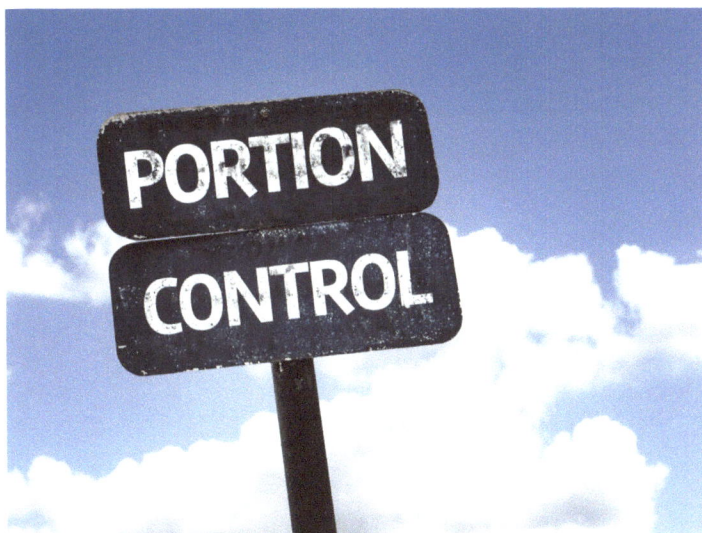

Day 7 Lifestyle Lesson:
20-50 chews per bite

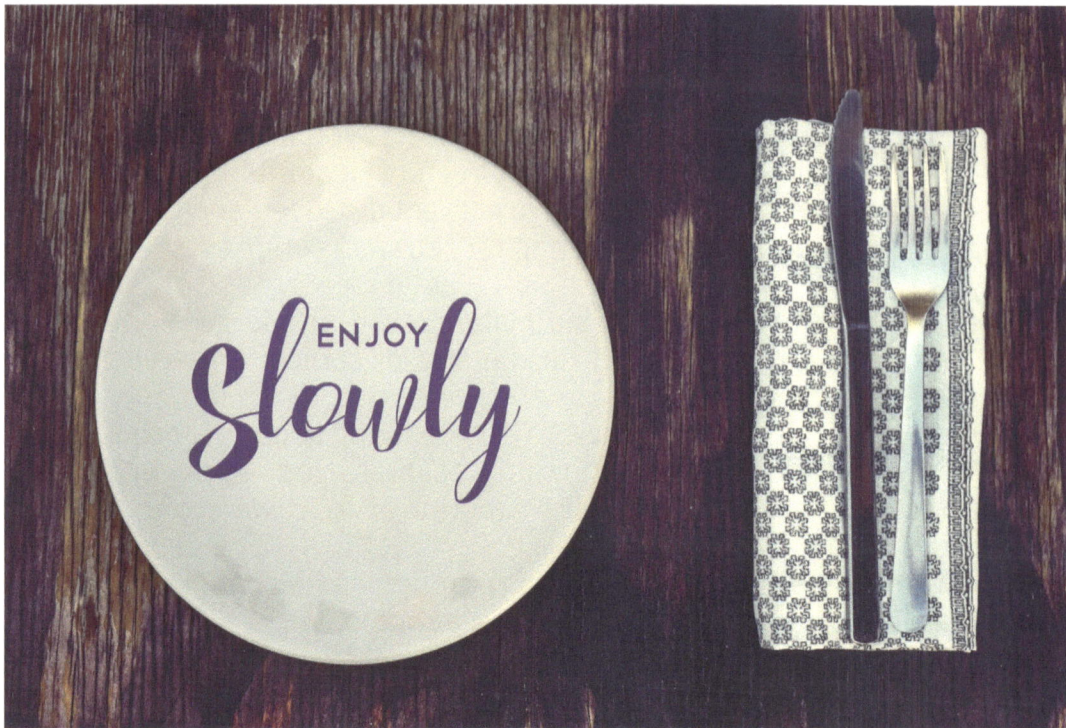

Our bodies are fearfully and wonderfully made. The complexity of the simple act of chewing is awe inspiring! The digestive process actually starts when we smell food, and then as we chew, we produce saliva and the process continues. Saliva contains digestive enzymes, so the longer you chew, the more time these enzymes have to start breaking down your food, making digestion easier on your stomach and small intestine. As we chew and swallow our food, the digestive tract starts to release hydrochloric acid which the stomach uses to break down our food into usable parts so that our body can absorb the nutrients. A study at Purdue University showed that chewing food longer allows nutrients to be utilized more efficiently, and there is a correlation between digestive efficiency and ideal weight. So how long should we chew our food? Horace Fletcher, a.k.a. "The Great Masticator," was a health figure in the 1800s who was famous for chewing each bite 100 times before swallowing. Most clinicians recommend 20-50 chews per bite as a fantastic starting place.

When in doubt, remember this, *your stomach does not have teeth*—so each bite needs to be liquefied before swallowing.

Day 7 Meals:
Refer to Chapter 10 Page

Day 7 Movement: 15-20 Minute Interval Walk
Refer to Chapter 9 Page

Day 8 Lifestyle Lesson:
Hara Hachi Bu

Okinawa is one of seven Blue Zones on the planet. These Blue Zones are infamous for housing the highest populations of healthy, active centenarians, or humans over one hundred years old! These superbly healthy Japanese have a saying that has kept them fit and shapely for centuries. Hara Hachi Bu means eat until 80% full. This advice is timeless and priceless! It is portion control in its truest form. This doesn't mean throw away 20% of your food. It means choose portions with your stomach leading the way and not with your eyes in control. If you would normally have two servings out of a dish, start with one serving instead. Eat slowly, focusing on those 20 to 50 chews per bite and tune into your level of hunger. You should leave the table with a comfortable feeling, not with a distended stomach or a belt that is now tight. It takes time (generally about twenty minutes) for your brain to signal to your stomach that you are full. So even if you don't feel 100% full when you stop eating, you will feel 100% full within twenty minutes.

EAT SLOWLY AND ENJOY YOUR FOOD

Day 8 Meals: **Refer to Chapter 10**

Day 8 Movement: 20-minute Strength Training
Refer to Chapter 9

Day 9 Lifestyle Lesson:
"Diet" and "Lite" = "Red Light"

On your health journey, you have probably consumed diet, lite, sugar-free, and fat-free products thinking you were doing your body good. And based on consumer marketing, who could blame you? The packages say "Healthy," "Whole Grain," and "Zero Calorie," and show healthy smiling models enjoying the product.

But research published in PLoS One, a scientific journal, showed that regular consumption of artificially sweetened soft drinks is associated with prediabetes, Type 2 Diabetes, and the complicated baggage like insulin resistance, impaired glucose intolerance, and belly fat that accompanies Type 2 Diabetes. In fact, it showed that drinking diet soda daily increased the risk of Type 2 Diabetes by 67%.

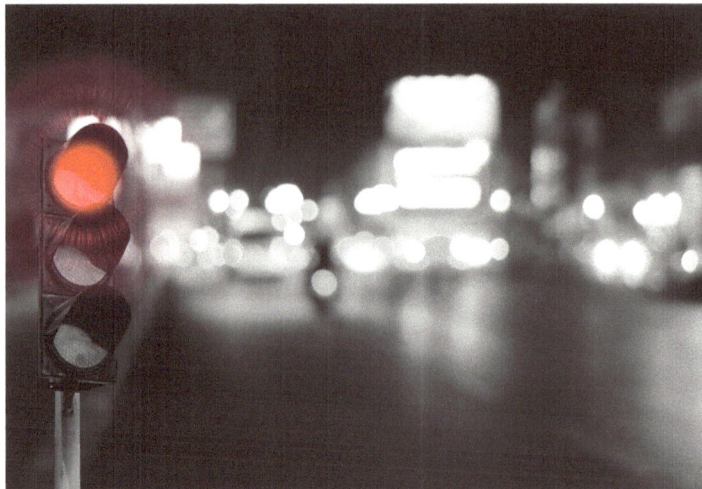

Wait a minute, did you have to re-read that?

The diet and lite versions, which are supposed to be great for Type 2 Diabetes, are the ones causing the problems!

I could bore you with mounds of research documents vilifying artificial sweeteners and flavors, but instead, I'm going to give you an avoid list. If the following ingredients are on the label, it is a RED LIGHT--WRONG WAY--ROAD CLOSED.

- Aspartame (Equal, NutraSweet)
- Sucralose (Splenda)
- Acesulfame Potassium (ACE K, Equal Spoonful, Sweet One, Sweet 'n Safe)
- Saccharin (Sweet 'N Low, Sweet Twin)

Day 9 Meals: **Refer to Chapter 10**

Day 9 Movement: 10 Minute H.I.I.T. Training
Refer to Chapter 9

Day 10 Lifestyle Lesson:
Red Zone vs.Green Zone

• Dr.Libby Weaver is an Australian Biochemist that has spoken extensively on how the function of the central nervous system should be considered when looking at weight loss and overall health. And clients in my practice have experienced drastic health changes after I taught them to understand and tap into their Green Zones and Red Zones. The central nervous system is comprised of the autonomic and the somatic nervous systems. The autonomic nervous system (ANS) controls visceral functions that occur below the level of consciousness and can be subdivided into the parasympathetic nervous system (PSNS) and the sympathetic nervous system (SNS).

• The Red Zone, or SNS, is our Speed and Greed zone. It is characterized by adrenaline, cortisol, sugar burning, and high-stress environments, and it is engaged through fear, stress, overload, caffeine, and excess glucose. Experts speak of "tigers chasing us in paleolithic times" to describe the effects of adrenaline, but that does not resonate in our lives today. We do not get chased by tigers, but our bodies do experience that same type of adrenaline and its aftermath. If your three-year-old granddaughter ran into a busy street you would run to save her without hesitation—this is your Red Zone in action. During adrenaline rushes and periods of high stress, your body shunts blood flow from the digestive system and sends it to your extremities, your arms and legs, so that you can run, jump, fight, or grab your three-year-old to save her life. But honestly how often do situations like this happen? Rarely! In this scenario, you tapped into your Red Zone; it served its purpose, and then you shifted back into the Green Zone as you watched the children play Ring Around the Rosie again. Chronic stress—like mounds of emails to read and respond to, trying to be superwoman and juggle sky high to-do lists—these types of stress tap into your Red Zone all day long! And the crux of how this plays into weight gain is that with chronic stress you never shift back into your Green Zone.

• The Green Zone, on the other hand, or PNS, is our Happy Place! It is our rest, digest, rebuild, and repair zone. It is characterized by fat burning, relaxation, and pleasure. It is engaged through diaphragmatic breathing, sleeping, and fueling with higher fat/ lower carb meals. Your body is only able to digest food when it is in the Green Zone and proper digestion parallels with ideal weight. It is only able to rebuild and repair from the day's activities and exercise when you sleep, and it is only able to burn your internal fat stores so you can lose weight when you are tapping into your Green Zone. Do you want to continue to live in the Red Zone or are you ready to shift into the Green Zone? The next three days of our Roadmap will go in depth on how to tap into your Green Zone to lose weight!

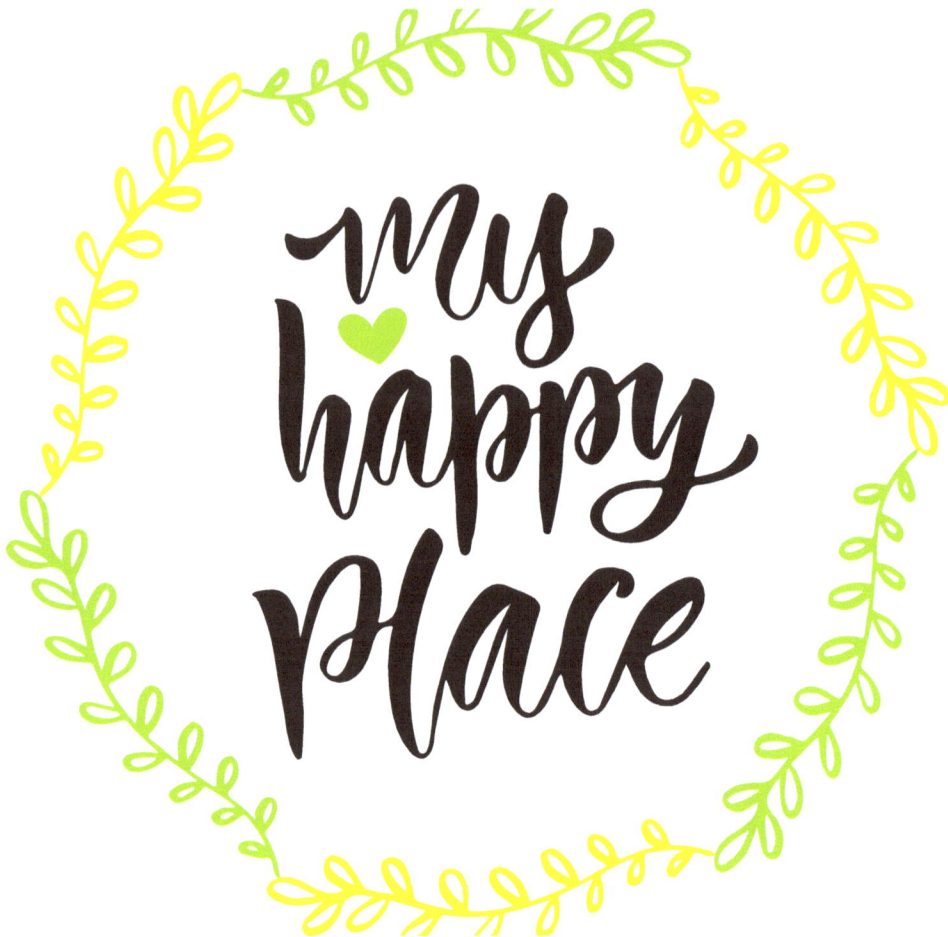

my ♥ happy place

Day 10 Meals: **Refer to Chapter 10**

Day 10 Movement: Gossip Walk
Refer to Chapter 9

Day 11 Lifestyle Lesson:
4-7-8 Breath

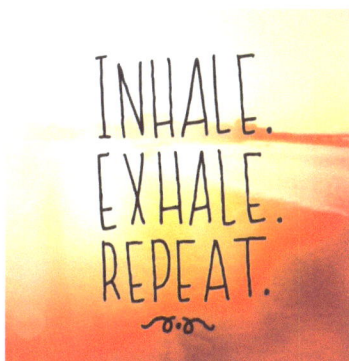

I call the Red Zone the "Speed and Greed Zone" since it monopolizes your body's efficiency. It greedily steals away the time your body needs to digest food which is the only means it has to turn nutrients into useable parts to rebuild and repair itself. The body cannot drop excess weight until it can rebuild and repair by efficiently digesting the nutrients you feed it. So how can we aid in this digestion process? By shifting into the Green Zone before eating and during any time of stress!

The 4-7-8 diaphragmatic breath technique was brought to mainstream culture by Harvard graduate Dr. Andrew Weil, MD. You can utilize this sub-60 second technique to upregulate the Green Zone before each meal and during times of stress to help lower cortisol and adrenaline. When you feel the volcano of stress rising, start the breath!

1. Place the tip of your tongue on the roof of your mouth, right behind your front teeth.
2. Breathe in through your nose for a count of 4.
3. Hold your breath for a count of 7.
4. Release your breath from your mouth with a whooshing sound for a count of 8.
5. Without a break, breathe in again for a count of 4, repeating the entire technique 3 to 4 times in a row, then resume normal breathing and activity.

https://www.drweil.com/videos-features/videos/breathing-exercises-4-7-8-breath/

Day 11 Meals: **Refer to Chapter 10**

Day 11 Movement: 20-minute Strength Training
Refer to Chapter 9

Day 12 Lifestyle Lesson:
Sleep the Pounds Away

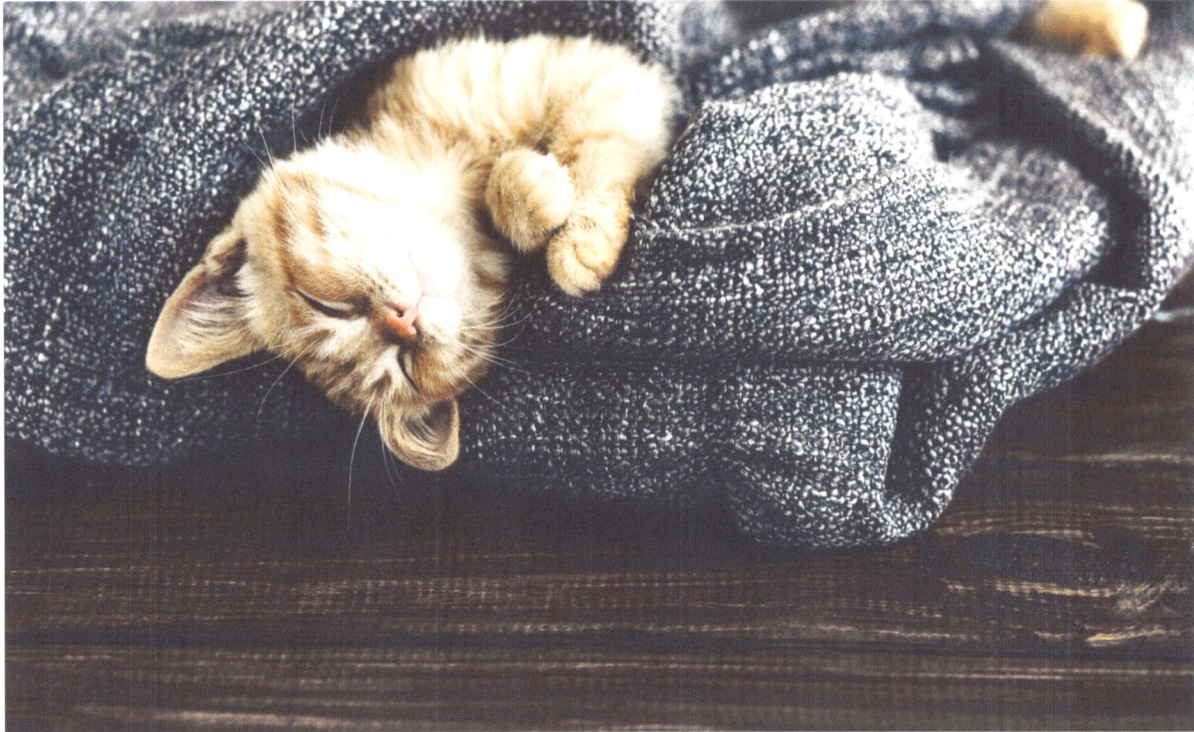

Just as appropriate exercise and snack choices influence fat loss, so does adequate sleep. Sleep provides a myriad of benefits for the body, especially for weight loss by tapping into the Green Zone.

1) Each time you exercise you tear down muscle fibers—which is perfect! Why? Because during sleep that muscle rebuilds better, stronger, and bigger than it was before. The equation is simply more exercise = more need for sleep. Bobby "Maximus" MacDonald was the training director for the movie, *300: Rise of an Empire*, a movie known for the chiseled bodies on the big screen. He required his actors-in-training to get eight to ten hours of sleep each night. Sleep plays such a pivotal foundation in body appearance that it was a requirement! You may not be training for a movie, but you are training for life, and if you do not get enough sleep your body will not be able to rebuild that muscle.

2) The body recovers from the emotional, psychological, and mental stress of the day during sleep. Hormones are released during sleep that help to regulate appetite control, stress, and metabolism.

3) Leptin, the satiety hormone, is reduced as sleep is reduced. Since leptin is a major player in appetite control and metabolism, having low levels of this hormone results

in increased cravings and a growing appetite. Trying to lose weight with inadequate leptin is akin to driving across the country with no gas stations. You will never make it!

4) If you suffer from low willpower, then increase your sleep to increase your willpower.

5) Remember, the secret to fat loss is to live in the Green Zone, and eight hours of sleep each night is one of the ways to cross over.

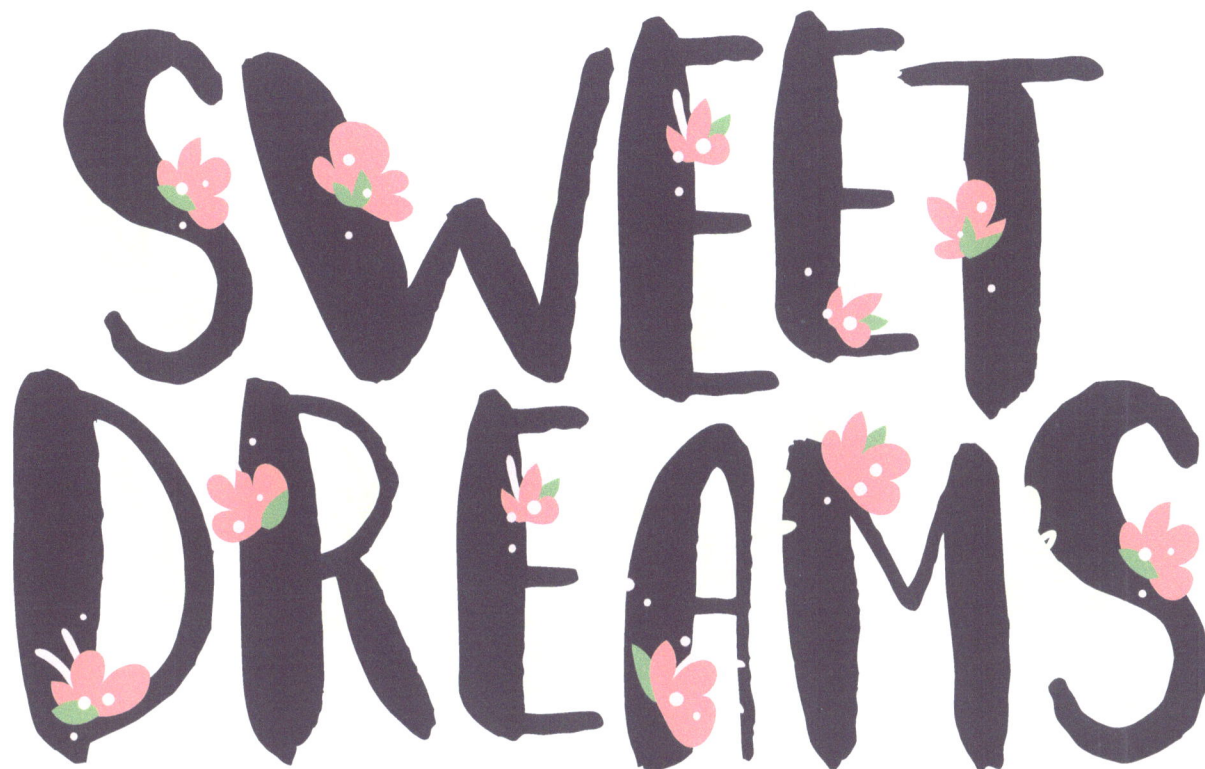

SWEET DREAMS

Day 12 Meals: **Refer to Chapter 10**

Day 12 Movement: **30-Minute Bubble Bath**

Day 13 Lifestyle Lesson:
Glucose Burning vs Fat Burning

Vehicles run on either diesel or gasoline, and if you have ever accidentally put diesel in your Tahoe you know full well the ramifications. Likewise, your body has access to two fuel sources: glucose (from carbohydrates and excess protein) and fat. Similarly, your body will either burn glucose or fat, but it will burn off the glucose before it can turn to the fat.

"Health and lifespan are determined by the proportion of fat versus sugar people burn throughout their lifetime. The more fat that one burns as fuel, the healthier the person will be, and the more likely they will live a long time. The more sugar a person burns, the more disease ridden and the shorter a lifespan a person is likely to have." -Dr. Ron Rosedale

Green Zone = fat burning zone (from your midsection!) Red Zone = sugar burning zone (fat gets stored since sugar gets burned)

How do I start burning fat instead of storing fat?

1) By reducing carbohydrate intake and increasing calories from fat we teach our bodies to use fat for fuel. Practice makes perfect. The longer you practice this 28-day meal plan and having a higher percent of your calories from fat sources, the better your body will become at burning internal fat for fuel.
2) By minimizing glucose in your bloodstream, your body can tap into your INTERNAL fat stores for fuel (a.k.a. burn off fat and lose weight).
3) Important tip—just adding fat to the equation will not work! The trick is to crowd out the glucose by focusing your plate on green leafy veggies, proteins, and fats. Removing foods like corn, grains, rice, potatoes, pasta, cookies, muffins, and bread is a must.
4) Our bodies maintain about 1 teaspoon of sugar in all 5 liters of our blood. Excess sugar in the blood must get metabolized or stored somewhere. If we struggle with insulin resistance (and are overweight) then our bodies will store that excess glucose as fat.
5) Just like sunflowers get energy from the sun and vehicles get energy from gasoline, our bodies require external energy in the form of calories. We are not focused on "burning" calories just like we don't try to "burn" off a tank of gasoline! Instead we want to increase calorie utilization efficiency by eating high fat/low carb meals.

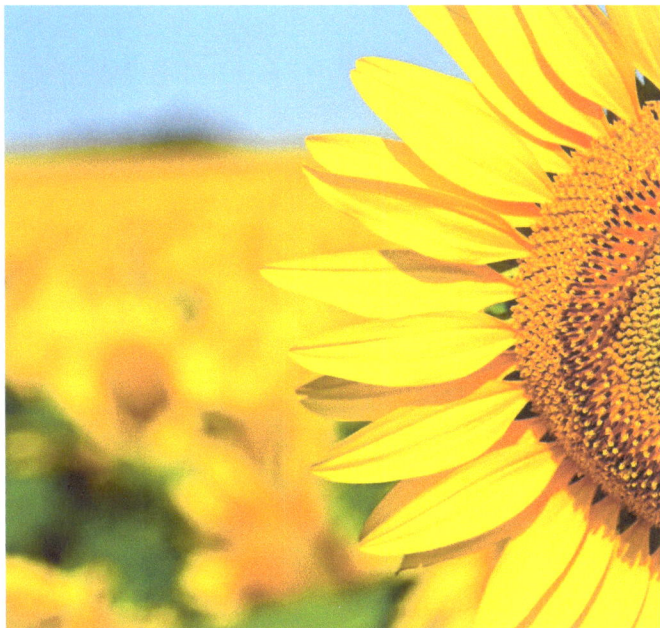

practice
MAKES
perfect

Day 13 Meals: **Refer to Chapter 10**

Day 13 Movement: 10 Minute H.I.I.T. Training
Refer to Chapter 9

Day 14 Lifestyle Lesson:
Week Two Check in and Re-Focus

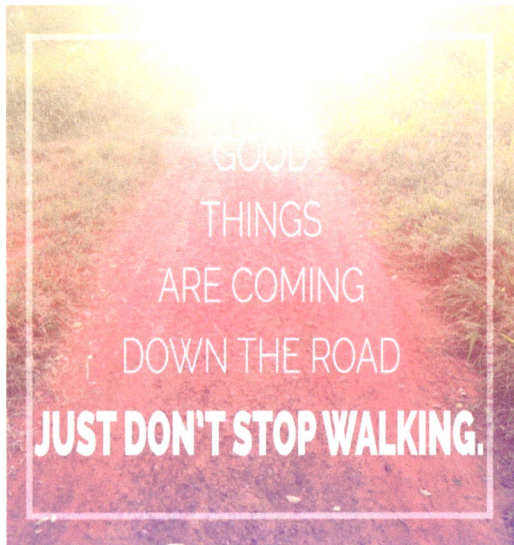

Congratulations!! You are halfway done with your health journey packing list. It is time to check in and course correct if necessary.

1) Now that you are allowing your Inner Siri to navigate, what choices and changes have you made? What new exercise can you tell is making a difference? What new food has become your favorite?

2) When you get a flat tire (nutritionally speaking), how do you respond? Write out a successful situation in which you paid for one flat tire instead of four. Kudos to you!

3) Are you chewing each bite 20-50 times? If not, why not? Now is the time to course correct and commit!

4) What strategies are you using to tap into your Green Zone? Which one has made the most noticeable difference? Have you tried using all three strategies in conjunction?

5) Are your clothes fitting differently? Do you have more energy? Do you feel more at peace and less stressed? Write out here what is new and good. Remember it so you can repeat it.

Day 14 Meals: **Refer to Chapter 10**

Day 14 Movement: 15-20 Minute Interval Walk
Refer to Chapter 9

Day 15 Lifestyle Lesson:
Love Yourself Today for Who You are Right Now, Not Where You Want to Be.

Grace amid Goals

These past two weeks I have loaded your car down with bags and boxes full of science and education. The next few days of packing will focus on more "feelings" and less "thinkings." Love yourself today. How many times do you say things like, "I'll be happy if I can lose twenty pounds." Or "I wish I still looked like I did in that picture on the mantle." Today is all you have. You can change tomorrow, but only by living out your goals with grace for your efforts today. Goals are priceless, but grace—not goals—gives way to abundance. Acknowledge with love that you are a work in progress on a health journey and that you are lovely today for where you are in your journey today. Grace amid goals feeds the body, mind, and spirit.

> GRATITUDE
> IS NOT ONLY THE GREATEST
> OF VIRTUES,
> BUT THE PARENT OF ALL OTHERS.

Day 15 Meals: **Refer to Chapter 10**

Day 15 Movement: 20-minute Strength Training
Refer to Chapter 9

Day 16 Lifestyle Lesson:
The Happy Marriage of Individual Will and Universal Law

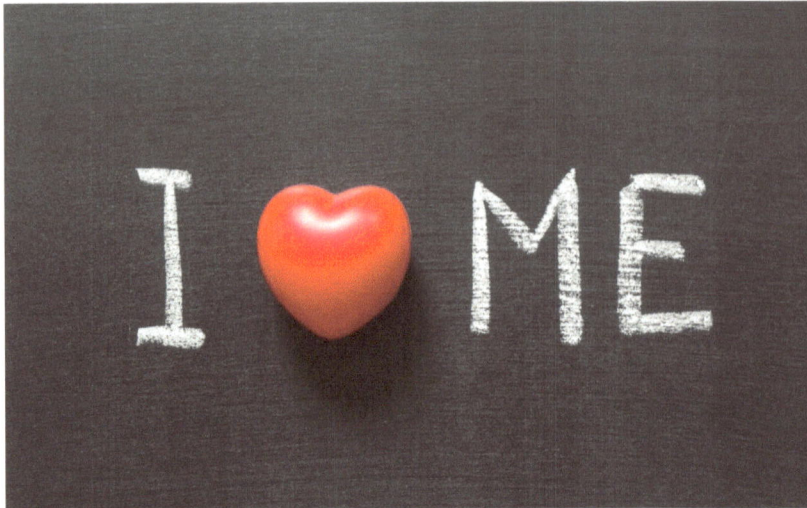

Society leads us to believe that if we put our best efforts and attention towards a goal, then we can accomplish anything; and if we fail, we must have done something wrong.

I have been 5'6" since the sixth grade, but I have a goal of being 5'9", so here is my action plan to accomplish this goal:

Stretch for an hour

Eat eight servings of string beans

Run four miles

Spend time concentrating on growing my bones

I could follow this regimen daily for the rest of my life, but will I ever be 5'9"? Did I do something wrong? Am I a failure?

I am all for "best efforts," "goal setting" and "striving for better." When it comes to our bodies I believe that all three aforementioned traits will catapult you along your Health Journey.

 BUT

There comes a time when we must look at what is realistic for our own bodies. Fitness looks different on everybody, so "striving for better" means a better version of you. Not a different you.

If your parents were large framed and of below average height, it doesn't matter how badly you want to have long lanky bones, it's just not in the cards you were dealt! This should be a very freeing sentiment: *never pressure yourself to look like someone else.*

When you realize that your Individual Will can put you in the position to meet the realistic goals within your Universal Law, then you have freed yourself from the baggage of comparison and guaranteed disappointment. Universal Law gave me a sturdy frame and potential for muscularity; it did not give me the option to be 5'9" with petite bones. There is no sense in me whining about it, wishing it would change, or hating myself for not accomplishing that desire.

If I am destined to be more of a crossfitter than a ballerina, then I am going to invest energy in being the best crossfitter I can and appreciate my friends who are ballerinas. Like me, when you focus your efforts and attention on being the best version of you, you are destined for success!

Day 16 Meals: **Refer to Chapter 10**

Day 16 Movement: 10 Minute H.I.I.T. Training
Refer to Chapter 9

Day 17 Lifestyle Lesson:
I Have a Choice; I am Not a Victim.

My body is a victim of my mouth.

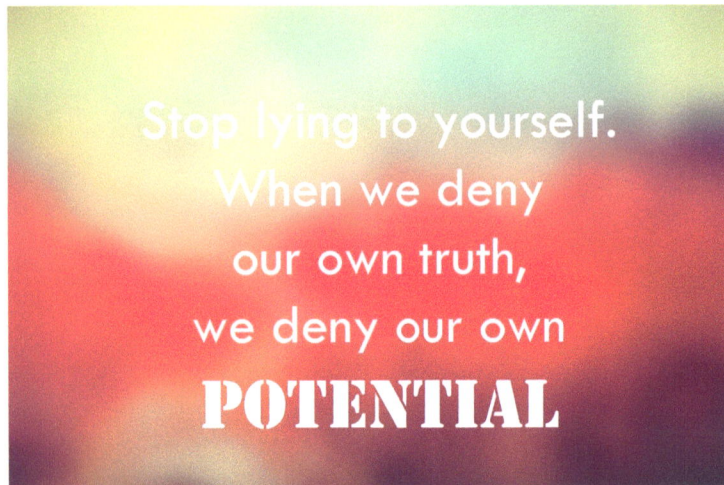

Stop lying to yourself. When we deny our own truth, we deny our own POTENTIAL

Your body does not hate you! It does not punish you by gaining weight, or by having joint pain, or by breaking out in rashes. Your body simply sits opposite your actions on a Cause and Effect Seesaw. If you spill red Kool-Aid down your shirt each day for a week, are you going to be mad at the shirt for becoming stained? Of course not! The shirt itself is the victim, not the perpetrator.

If you want the red stain to go away you will go through two important steps:

1) Stop spilling Kool-Aid.
2) Apply stain removal and wash the shirt.

You will first stop the action (spilling Kool-Aid) that is causing the symptom (red stain.) Then you will apply measures (stain removal and washing) to salvage the shirt. Just to drive the lesson home, let me spell out the link between the shirt and your body. If you continuously eat processed food and diet sodas your body will become stained with excess fat.

Common sense tells us you do not need a pill to lessen the effects of spilling the Kool-Aid. You need to quit spilling the Kool-Aid. This is tough love ladies, but you must stop filling your body with junk.

Step two is to clean up the mess. Your body needs some TLC through nourishing movement, healing foods, and proper hydration and sleep. Apply some stain remover, wash your shirt, and now the Cause and Effect Seesaw will lead to weight loss and health gain.

Day 17 Meals: **Refer to Chapter 10**

Day 17 Movement: Gossip Walk
Refer to Chapter 9

Day 18 Lifestyle Lesson:
Quiet the Inner Child

"I want the chocolate cake! Everyone else here is having it. This is not fair! I don't know why they can have cake and I can't." Are these thought bubbles from a 3-year-old or from you? I can assure you my thought bubbles can look more like a toddler's than a 30-something's when I am faced with chocolate chip brownies! Let's face it ladies, food desires and restrictions can turn us into toddlers in the blink of an eye. How do you mitigate the "food wantings" temper tantrum? The same way you teach a toddler to cease her tantrums.

1) Go outside of the moment and think as a mother seeing the bigger picture.

a. You mothered your child with patience and intellect, seeing the bigger picture. When your 3-year-old wanted to run from one end of the pool to the other you stopped her. You realized she would likely slip and fall hard on that wet concrete and end up with a knocked-out tooth, bloody nose, or both. She does not care about those possibilities or even realize the danger. But as the mother, you know it is in her best interest, even if it makes her angry, to prevent that possible fall.

b. When you fall into "wantings," stop and use the 4-7-8 breath and then think outside of the moment. Look at the bigger picture: is this "wanting" going to serve your purpose of losing weight or is it going to give you a knocked-out tooth and bloody nose? A 3-year-old rushing to the other end is no different than you rushing into a slice of cake. Allow the mother inside of you to speak rationally about the situation. You are not deprived; you do not earn cake or deserve cake. You deserve to meet your goals.

2) Don't give in to the tantrum.

a. I just witnessed a poor young mother in the store with a red-faced toddler screaming loudly for a bag of M&Ms. At first, the mother tried to redirect her little boy, but as the decibels of his screaming increased she gave in and gave up. He immediately stopped the fit as he wrapped his little hands around the bag. And I have no doubt he learned a lesson—the next time he wants a bag of candy he will use this same tactic again.

b. The inner child in your brain will be screaming at you to give her the pint of ice cream. Resist! Distract yourself with something else! If you are at home when the fit starts then put in a load of laundry, or go water the flower pots outside. If you are at a store, move on to the next aisle. Only buy what was on your list. Don't give in and give up. You are worth more than an "I give up," and you deserve to meet your goals.

3)   Reward positive behaviors.

a. Self-discipline is self-love. You know that guilt that follows an impulsive indulgence that you did not intend to happen? It's like a black hole! The regret, remorse, and negative self-talk aftermath are nauseating. Reward yourself before you indulge. For example, tell yourself that if you do not have the ice cream right now, that you will allow yourself to have a scoop of it tomorrow. That gives you distance, space, and time to buffer the impulse. You are not saying "NO!" You are saying "Not right now!" Tomorrow, if you still want the scoop of ice cream, then you have planned for it and you can rearrange your snack choices all day to account and budget for it. This is an act of self-love. When you use self-discipline, you avoid the guilt that follows impulsive decisions.

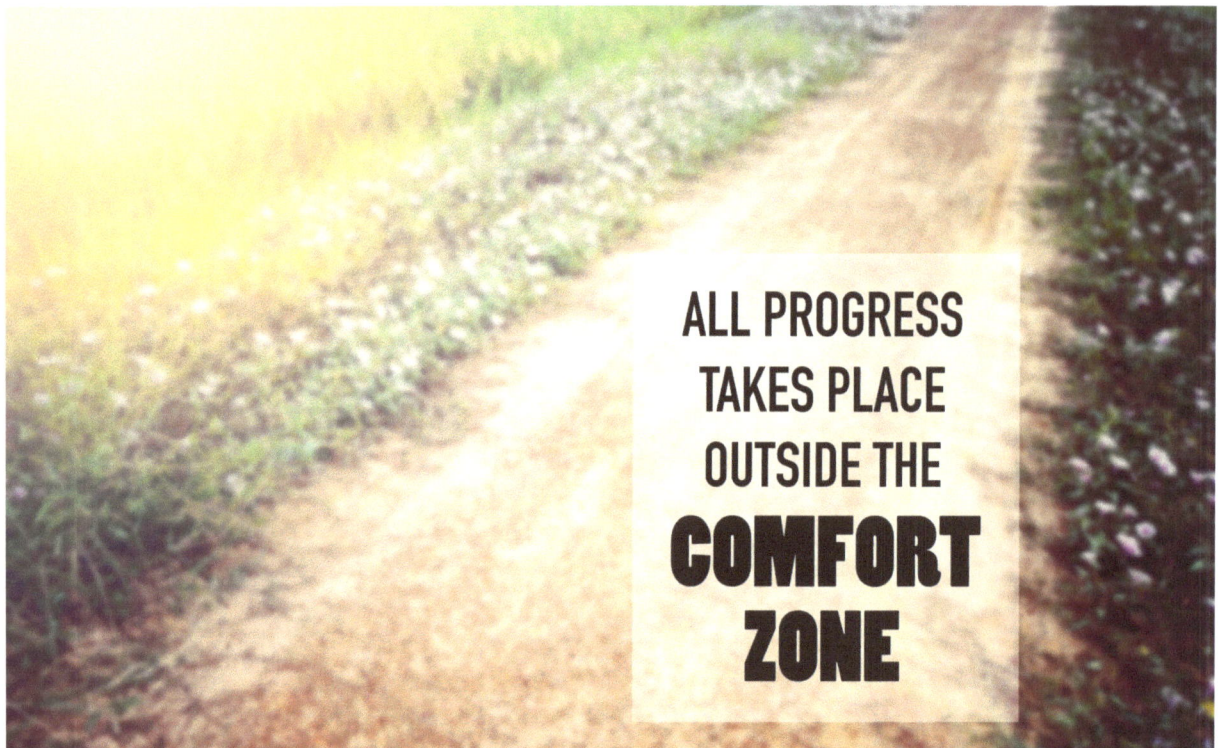

Day 18 Meals: **Refer to Chapter 10**

Day 18 Movement: 20-minute Strength Training
Refer to Chapter 9 Page

Day 19 Lifestyle Lesson:
Get a Plate—Avoid the Hate

Although I was tempted to put this as the Lifestyle Lesson for Day 1, I chose to put it here with just a little over a week left of your journey. Since you are healing your body through nutritious meals and healing movement, many of you will have already put aside this self-sabotaging behavior. If you still notice an urge to grab a spoon and dig in or take the bag of almonds to your desk, then it's time to teach you a trick.

Eating impulsively is Self-Sabotage. When you eat out of a bag or dish you:

1) Lose track of the volume of food and over consume.

2) Swallow while only chewing 4-5 times.

3) Miss out on the tastes and qualities of the food.

Food is fun! We should enjoy it not inhale it.
When you are tempted to grab a fork and even out the pan of brownies or sit in the pantry munching on an open container while deciding what to eat, admit that you are sabotaging yourself. Say it out loud, "Get a plate—avoid the hate." That quick little reminder will cue you to pour your snack onto a plate or bowl.

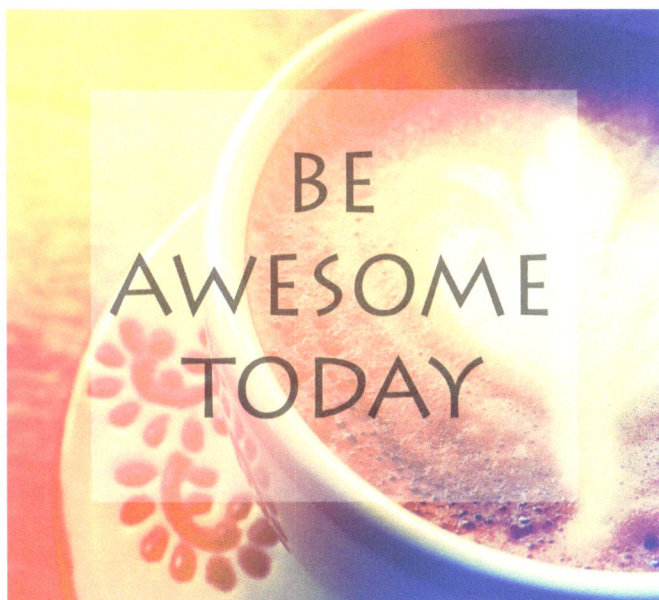

BE AWESOME TODAY

Day 19 Meals: **Refer to Chapter 10**

Day 19 Movement: **30 Minute Bubble Bath**

Day 20 Lifestyle Lesson:
Passeggiata!

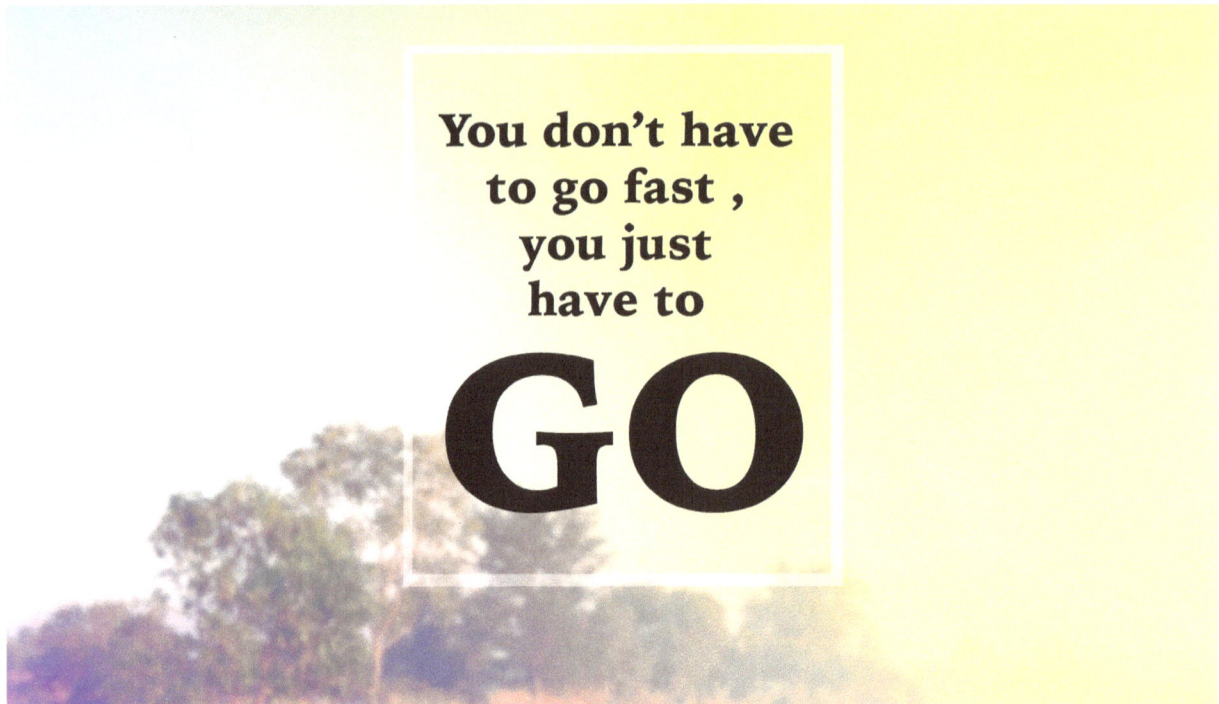

You don't have to go fast, you just have to GO

Recent studies have shown the Italian custom of slow social strolls in the evening significantly improves blood sugar levels in those with pre-diabetes and Type 2 Diabetes. Just like the 4-7-8 breath and the 20-50 chews per bite, this is another completely free course correction method! After dinner put on your walking shoes, grab the fam, and head down the street. No sweat involved, no intervals, no stopwatches—this is a relaxing and rejuvenating way to tap into your Green Zone and aid digestion. Listen to the birds and chat about the day.

Implemented with routine, three to four times per week, Passeggiata is one of the simplest and most effective tools on your health journey packing list.

Day 20 Meals: **Refer to Chapter 10**

Day 20 Movement: 10 Minute H.I.I.T. Training
Refer to Chapter 9

Day 21 Lifestyle Lesson:
Food for Thought

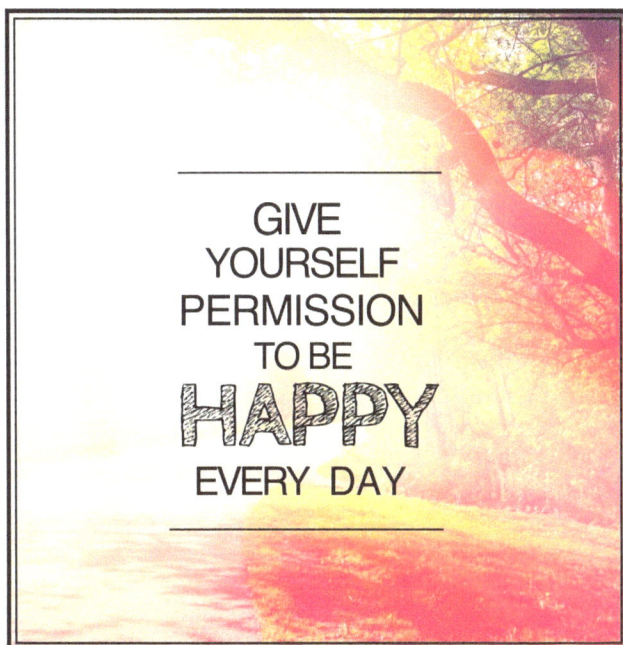

GIVE YOURSELF PERMISSION TO BE HAPPY EVERY DAY

Three weeks in and you are on the home stretch! We have just one week of packing left before you drive off into the sunset! Today I am giving you a list of thoughts, ideas, and sayings to add to your bucket of "thinkings" and "feelings" from the past twenty days.

1) Nourishment as gratification. Focus your intentions on being gratified through nutritious choices, not on gratifying your taste buds with sugar fixes. What does this mean to you?

2) Make an Excessive list. Where are you excessive in your life? I personally can list these three: busyness, chocolate, and exercise. Bodies and minds seek homeostasis. If you can target areas in your life that you exhibit excessiveness in and search to balance them you will see a positive reaction in your body because the body houses stress. When I set my alarm for 4:15 am and train fitness clients until noon, then counsel diabetes patients until 4 pm, then get home and check food logs for my online clients until 6 pm, then cook dinner and spend time with my family until bedtime, I am setting myself up for burnout and anxiety overload. The same holds true when I train for long-distance triathlon and spend twenty hours each week swimming, biking, running, and lifting weights. I fall face first into brownies when these facets of my life get out of balance. Then the guilt cycle begins! Here is the magic formula that worked for my particular situation:

a) I have learned to limit the number of clients I take during the day.
b) I budget two hours for online coaching only on Thursdays.
c) I keep my weekends sacred: no work, only fun and family.
d) I gave up long distance triathlons and now limit my exercise to five days per week.

These lifestyle changes have completely erased my sugar cravings.

Write out your "Excessive" list here. What small changes can you implement to bring you more balance?

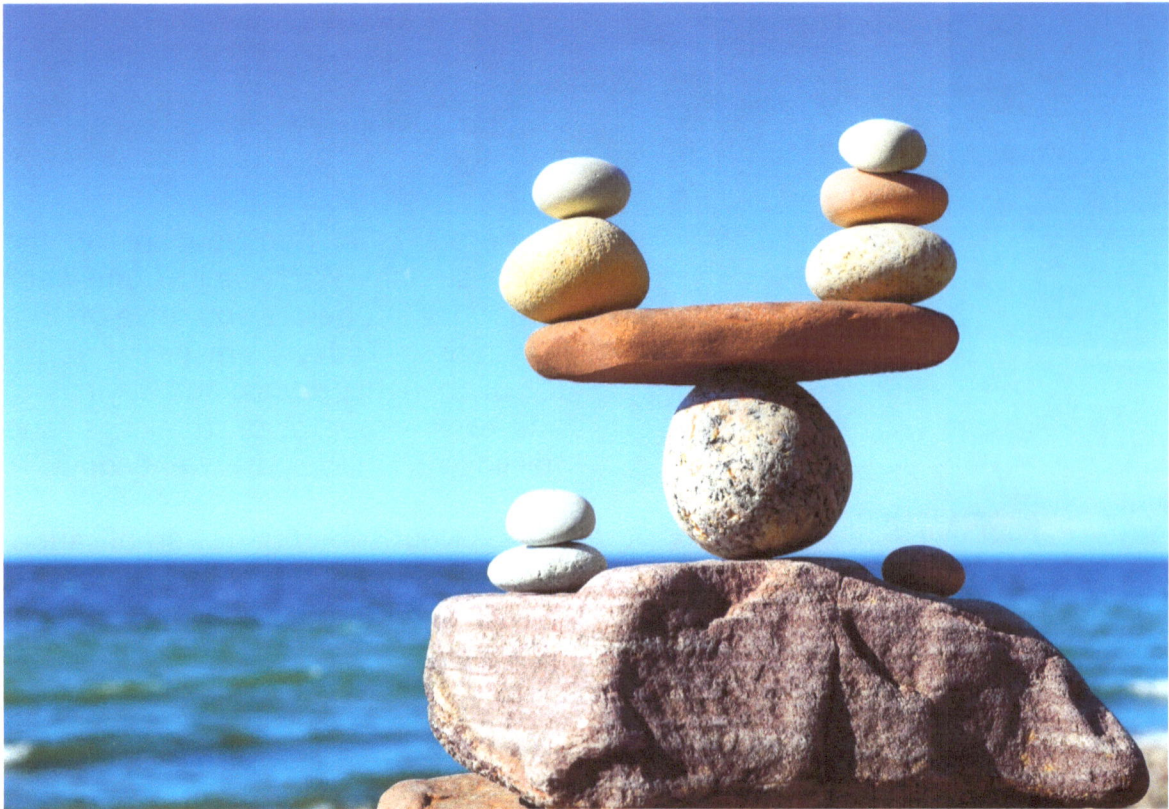

3) Strive for "Happier not Happiness." Being happy is a conscious choice—an act of being, not an emotion. Just like Tigger and Eeyore, you can choose to be happy with the rain clouds or not. This statement is not to minimize depression or valleys on our journey like deaths and divorces. It is just to point out that you have a choice. Rain clouds can dampen your spirit, but they can't take away your choice. Becoming happier is in your reach. Happiness, on the other hand, is elusive and ambiguous. Instead of reaching "Happiness" when you are 30 pounds less, focus on choosing to be Happier when you drink bulletproof coffee instead of that grande mocha latte. Happy people are shown to have healthier habits which lead to healthier lives.

What are three things in your life today that you can choose to be happy about?
1) _____ 2) _____ 3) _____
Gretchen Rubin is my favorite expert on how to strive for Happier not Happiness.
http://gretchenrubin.com/

Day 21 Meals: **Refer to Chapter 10**

Day 21 Movement: 15-20 Minute Interval Walk
Refer to Chapter 9 Page

Day 22 Lifestyle Lesson:
Say NO to Water Anorexia

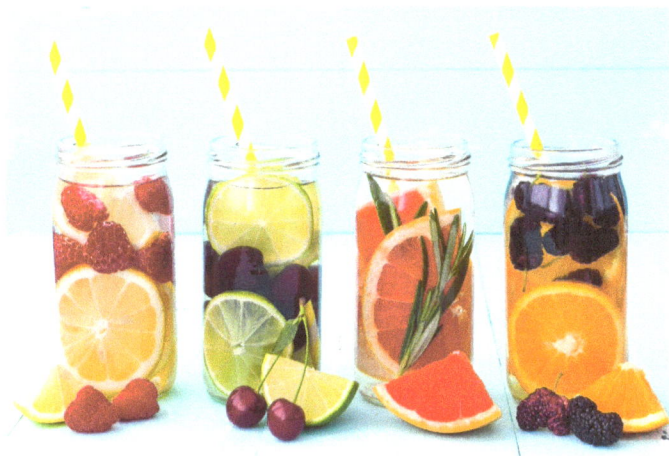

I want water to be the first item you pack on your health journey—quite literally! I will be bold enough to say that you will never reach your weight loss goals if you do not commit to increased water intake. Don't like water? Get over it! That sounds harsh, but seriously ladies, if you are battling sugar cravings, headaches, blood sugar crashes, and fatigue, then honor your body and give it the water it is craving. Water flows through the blood, carrying oxygen and nutrients to cells and flushing wastes out of our bodies. It cushions our joints and soft tissues. Without water as a routine part of our intake, we cannot digest or absorb food. There is an understanding of how harmful anorexia is to the body, but have you considered how refusal to drink water affects your body? Humans can live weeks without food but only days without water. It's a big deal!

Rules of the Road:

- Drink 16 ounces every morning before you eat or leave the house. Give your liver some love with my Liver Lover morning water concoction!
- Drink half of your bodyweight in ounces of water each day.
- Spread your water intake evenly throughout the day instead of water loading. Drinking all of your water in one or two settings is like flooding the daffodils before your two-week vacation instead of having a sprinkler timing system in place.
- Add eight ounces of water for every thirty minutes of exercise and every four ounces of alcohol.

Buy yourself a cute Yeti, Tervis, or a pretty glass container that you can take water all day long with you. At a convenience store a plastic water bottle is $0.89 and sweet tea is $1.79, so the $20 water container would pay for itself in a month! If you constantly have fresh cold water within arm's grasp you are less tempted to yearn for sodas and teas. In the past three years, four clients have given me water containers with my initials, favorite colors, or triathlon symbols on it. They see me carrying my water and refilling it constantly, day in and day out. Here are a few reasons why I view water as the most important staple on your health journey:

1) Research reports have shown a 44% greater rate of weight loss among water group participants compared to non-water participants over a 12-week randomized controlled trial.
2) Another study showed that after drinking approximately 17 ounces of water, the

subjects' metabolic rates—or the rate at which calories are burned—increased by 30%.

DEHYDRATING DRINKS

• Coffee, tea, soda, alcohol, and energy drinks are not water.
• These drinks contain water, but also contain dehydrating agents.

Signs of too much water

• Disrupted sleep-waking every few hours to urinate.
• Mineral imbalance—this would be picked up on bloodwork from your physician.

Signs of too little water/dehydration

• Fatigue
• Hunger
• Headaches
• Sugar cravings

I have never heard an excuse that I condoned for not drinking water. If you cannot remember to drink water, then set a timer on your phone. Every ten minutes you should take two big gulps of water. If you are a teacher, then plan to drink ¼ of your water before school, ¼ at lunch, ¼ after school, and ¼ in the evening. I was a third-grade teacher for three years—yes, it is more of a struggle for you, but you can do it!

Tip to jazz up your water: Use infused water for flavor and variety!
Chop up about one cup of your favorite fruit and add to a gallon of water.
Allow the fruit flavors to infuse for twenty minutes.
Pour infused water into your new special water container!
You can refill the gallon for two days before throwing out the fruit and starting again.
Favorite combos:
1) cucumber and mint
2) watermelon and apple
3) berry medley
4) orange, lemon, and lime

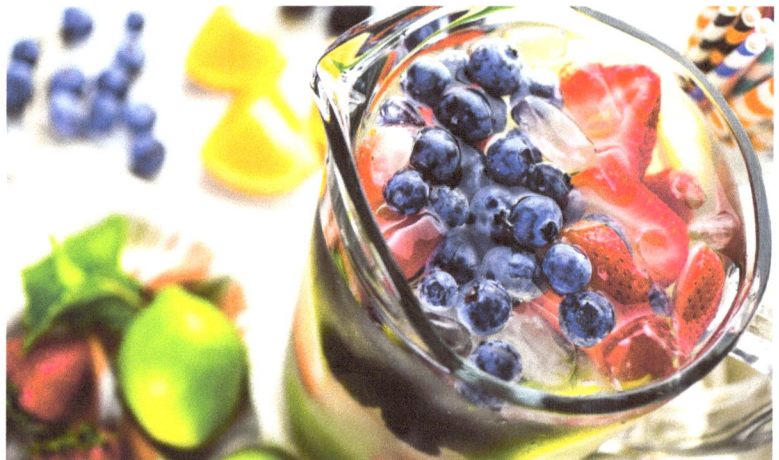

Day 22 Meals: **Refer to Chapter 10**

Day 22 Movement: 20-minute Strength Training
Refer to Chapter 9

Day 23 Lifestyle Lesson:
Kill the Sugar Monster!

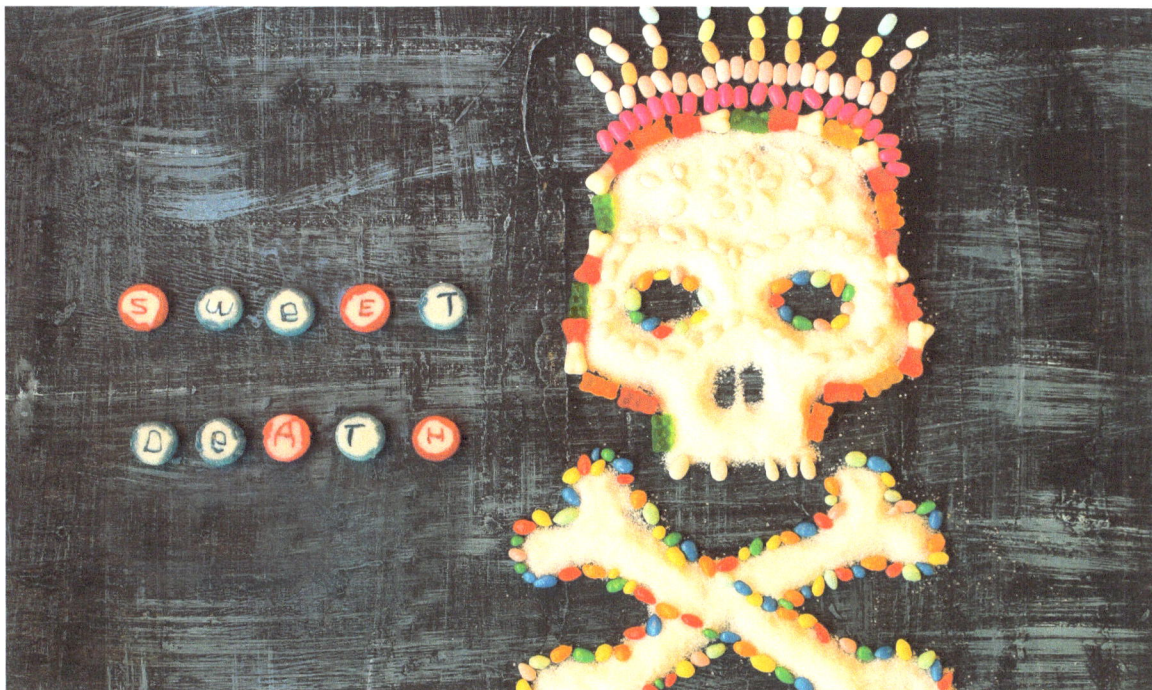

Most of my patients with Type 2 Diabetes battle sugar cravings. Not all of them were addicted to sweet tea and sodas, but 100% of the patients addicted to sweet tea and sodas do report sugar cravings. The next item on your packing list is my foolproof solution to reducing soda and sweet tea addictions in four to six weeks without going cold turkey. I have had patients reduce sugar intake by two hundred grams or more per day, just through reducing sports drinks, sweet teas and sodas! Some have lost over thirty pounds in a month just by following this system.

1) Sweet Tea Reduction: If you are used to buying a 44-ounce convenience store cup every day of the week then keep doing it! If you are used to buying a 32-ounce cup then stick to that size; you will progress faster through the process. Also, if you only indulge in sweet tea occasionally, then for the love of butter don't follow my suggestions on daily use! The goal is to meet you where you are and slide it down to unsweet tea with as little pain as possible. We are going to make small changes each week that have large scale cumulative effects. My intent is for the change to be subtle enough that you notice but do not detest the difference. We are retraining your taste buds day by day!

Week 1: For every drink purchase: 44-ounce cup of ¾ sweet tea and ¼ unsweet tea with lots of ice! Sip slowly through the straw. Savor the flavor (water is the only thing you are allowed to gulp!)

Week 2: For every drink purchase: 32-ounce cup of ¾ cup sweet tea and ¼ unsweet tea with lots of ice! Sip slowly through the straw. Savor the flavor (water is the only thing you are allowed to gulp!)

Week 3: For every drink purchase: 32-ounce cup of ½ sweet tea and ½ unsweet tea with lots of ice! Sip slowly through the straw. Savor the flavor (water is the only thing you are allowed to gulp!)

Week 4: For every drink purchase: 22-ounce cup of ¼ sweet tea and ¾ unsweet tea with lots of ice! Sip slowly through the straw. Savor the flavor (water is the only thing you are allowed to gulp!)

Week 5: For every drink purchase: 22-ounce cup of 100% unsweet tea with lots of ice! Sip slowly through the straw. Savor the flavor (water is the only thing you are allowed to gulp!)

Week 6: Now your goal is to increase water and reduce unsweet tea consumption. If you were used to getting tea every day, switch to every other day. After that becomes second nature, cut it down to just one per week, then one every other week, then one per month till you no longer miss it!

Note: Unsweet tea does not have to be completely eliminated. Just please be sure you are not choosing unsweet tea as a replacement for water!

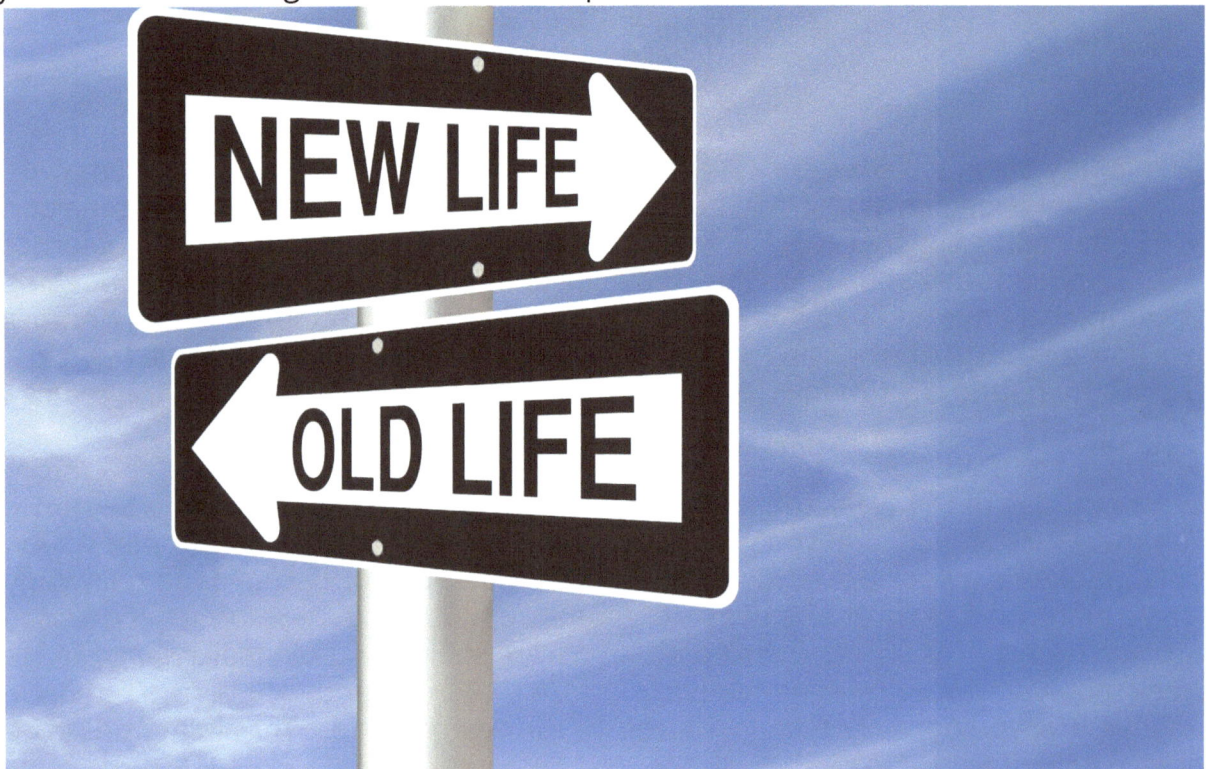

2) Soda/Diet Soda reduction: We are going through the same process as with the sweet tea reduction with the goal of completely eliminating all sodas and diet sodas forever. Remember Diet = Red Light. They have zero nutritional value and in fact, are correlated to the extra fat and inflammation burdening you. If you can go cold turkey then please do! The faster you eliminate all sodas and diet sodas, the faster you will shed belly fat.

Week 1: For every drink purchase: 44-ounce cup of poison (soda) with lots of ice! Sip slowly through the straw. As soon as you are done, brush your teeth. You do not need the sugar monster hanging out on your tongue and demanding more sugar. Be prepared to have to stand strong against cravings. The chemical composition is engineered to induce cravings to make you buy more!

Week 2: For every drink purchase: 32-ounce cup of poison (soda) lots of ice! Sip slowly through the straw. As soon as you are done, brush your teeth. You do not need the sugar monster hanging out on your tongue and demanding more sugar. Be prepared to have to stand strong against cravings. The chemical composition is engineered to induce cravings to make you buy more!

Week 3: For every drink purchase: 22-ounce cup of poison (soda) with lots of ice! Sip slowly through the straw. As soon as you are done, brush your teeth. You do not need the sugar monster hanging out on your tongue and demanding more sugar. Be prepared to have to stand strong against cravings. The chemical composition is engineered to induce cravings to make you buy more!

Week 4: Only purchase half the number of sodas. For example, if you have been having one 22-ounce soda daily, now go to every other day. If you were having three 22-ounce drinks every day, now have only one 22-ounce daily.

Week 5: Halve the number of sodas again. For example, if you have been having one 22-ounce drink daily, now go to every other day. After that becomes second nature, cut it down to just one per week, then one every other week, then one per month until you no longer miss it!

Now your goal is to increase water and eliminate all soda consumption. Once you have eliminated the garbage, never add it back!

Day 23 Meals: **Refer to Chapter 10**

Day 23 Movement: 10 Minute H.I.I.T. Training
Refer to Chapter 9

Day 24 Lifestyle Lesson:
I am What I Eat Today

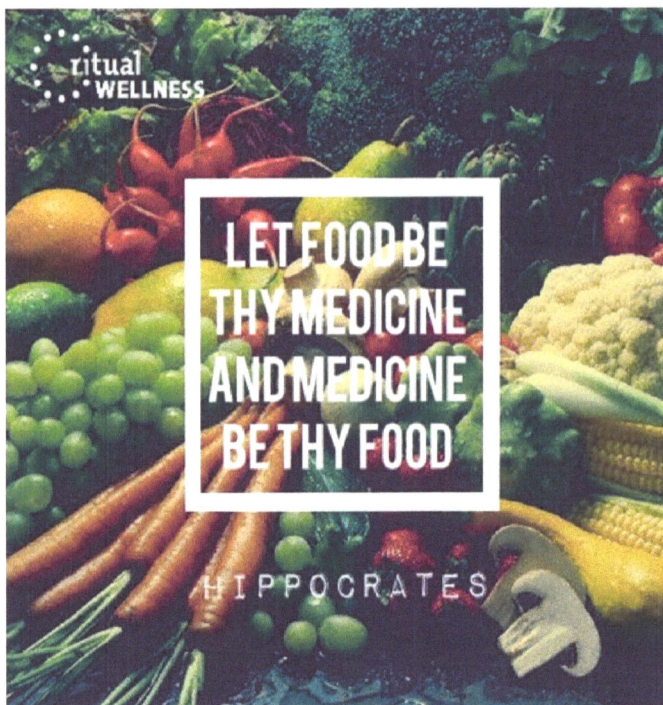

LET FOOD BE THY MEDICINE AND MEDICINE BE THY FOOD

HIPPOCRATES

After a nine-day trip to Turks and Caicos, I returned to my life as a health and wellness coach about ten pounds heavier, with a huge ganglion cyst in my wrist, with eczema, and so swollen my socks left imprints! Even though I ate in quality restaurants the effects of MSG (see Chapter 5 for more information) left battle scars on my body. To cleanse my body and get rid of the damage I caused from the processed food, I started journaling every day with the intent of seeing how my cellular health would repair in three months. I realized, based on the lifespan of cells, that this would not be an overnight transformation. But I also realized that in just 90 days many of my damaged cells would be replaced with brand new healthy ones. I was literally changing my body each day based on the foods I ate. Here are some of my journal pages:

June 23rd In 3 months, my body will be made of: quinoa, zucchini, apple, kombucha, chicken, romaine, macadamias, balsamic vinegar, almond butter, carrots, olive oil, turkey, avocado, spinach, red onions, sesame seeds. 100oz water

On days like this I was thrilled at the thought of how healthy my body would be in the next 90 days. But there were also days that looked like this:

July 3rd In 3 months, my body will be made of: coffee, coconut oil, cacao butter, brisket, BBQ sauce, spinach, homemade roll, chocolate cake, broccoli, homemade ranch, pizza-lots, chocolate chip cookie-3, 65oz water

I used this journaling method to keep me accountable. I knew I would not be perfect everyday—that is unrealistic and impractical. But when I started realizing that I literally am what I eat, it helped me clean it up after splurges to stay on track for 90 days.

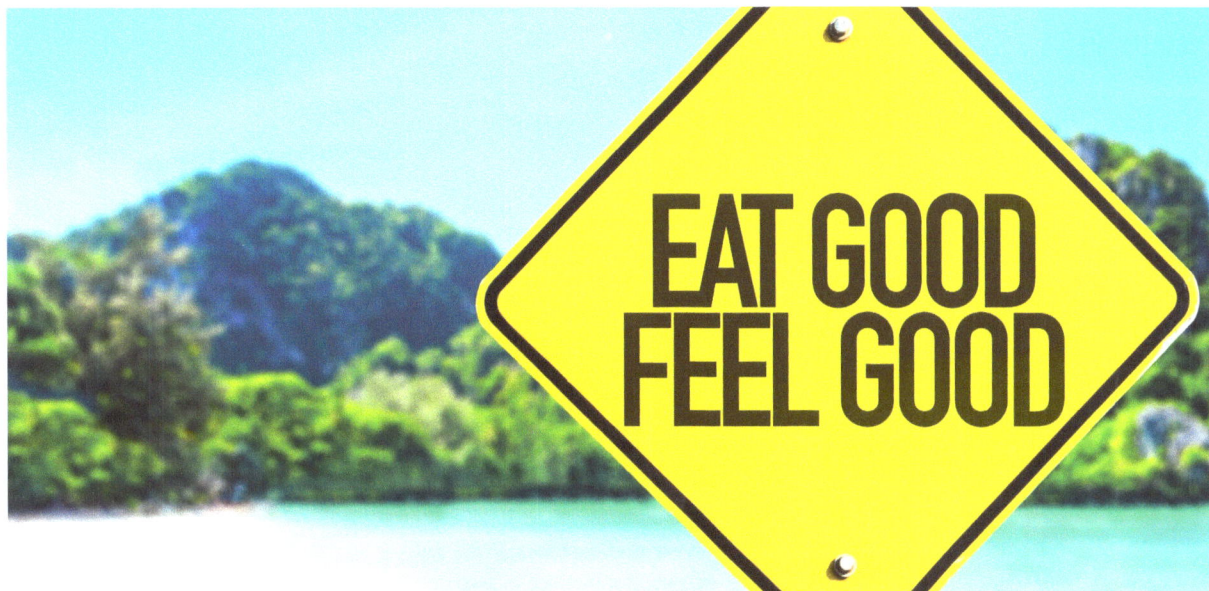

Here is a chart to show you the average cell turnover rate:

Taste buds	10 days
Red blood cells	4 months
White blood cells	2-5 days
Liver cells	6 months-1 year
Colon cells	4 days
Small intestine	2-4 days
Stomach	2-9 days
Lungs alveoli	8 days
Platelets	10 days
Skin cells	10-30 days
Fat cells	8 years

Day 24 Meals: **Refer to Chapter 10**

Day 24 Movement: Gossip Walk
Refer to Chapter 9

Day 25 Lifestyle Lesson:
I am What I Eat Today

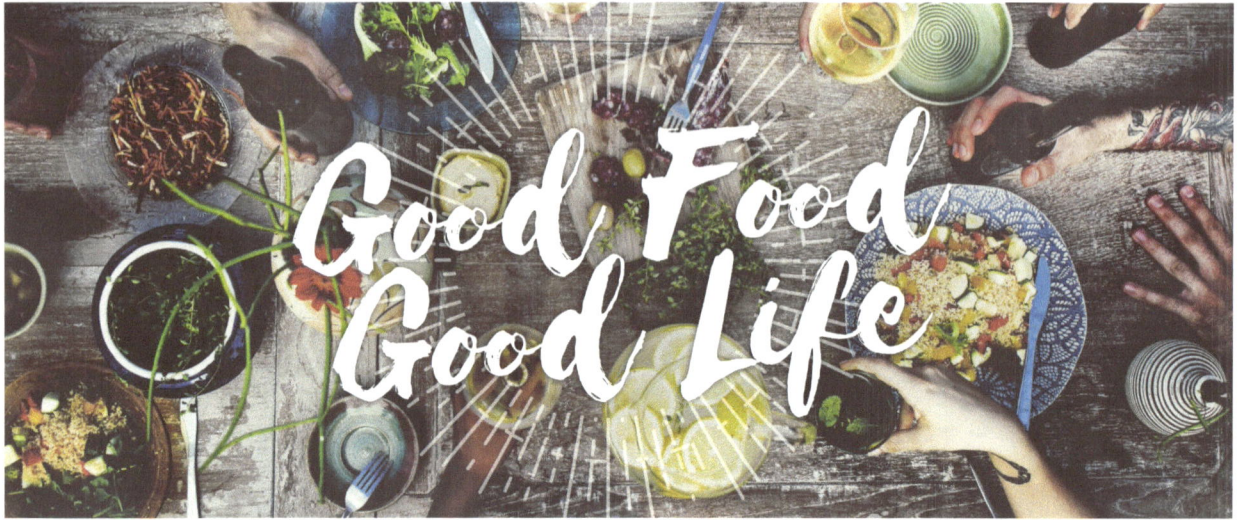

1. Will Durant—"We are what we repeatedly do. Excellence then, is not an act but a habit."
2. Albert Einstein—The definition of insanity is when we do the same thing over and over again and expect different results.
3. Ralph Waldo Emerson—We are what we eat (paraphrased).

Ponder these three sayings for a moment. Say them again in your head, but where you see a "we" replace it with a "me" or an "I."

What are the two common denominators in all three quotes?   Repetition and Me!
The stuff you put in and on your body is the #1 influence you have on your body. To make the largest scale impact on your body, you must alter the way you touch your body through food. Our bodies transport us through millions of microbes, bacterium, smells, chemicals, and toxins each day. The body is a brilliant vehicle, and it has two major interfaces with the world.

A) Skin
B) Digestive tract (the food that comes in).

Your food choices need to serve your purpose.

Day 25 Meals:**Refer to Chapter 10**

Day 25 Movement: 20-minute Strength Training
Refer to Chapter 9

Day 26 Lifestyle Lesson:
Empty House

Move your Body

Have you noticed that houses on the market start to fall apart after they have been empty for a couple months? A shingle here and there tears off, tiles curl up, and doors start to hang unevenly. A body without movement is like a house without people. Bodies were designed for movement. Sitting in cars all day or in office cubicles removes the body from its natural environment.

According to Tommy Wood, MD, Ph.D., at Nourish Balance Thrive, learning to sit less and take regular movement breaks will help you on your quest to improve blood sugar control.

No doubt many of you have tried 45 minutes of elliptical, bike, or treadmill hoping to drop some pounds just to be disappointed with minimal progress. A recent study geared to participants with Type 2 Diabetes instructed them to "replace approximately 5 hours per day of sitting with 2 hours of walking and 3 hours of standing. Participants were instructed to break up their sitting time, preferably every 30 min, by dividing the walking/standing activities into smaller bouts over the day."

The outcome showed that breaking sitting with standing and light-intensity walking improved glucose levels and insulin sensitivity to a greater extent than 60 minutes of structured exercise! Our Movement Map follows this same protocol. Move a little, often! According to Dr. Wood, adding movement "snacks" throughout the day is one of the simplest ways to improve health. Starting today, set your timer on your smartphone for 30 minutes and take a movement snack for five minutes. You'll return to your task with increased blood flow for greater clarity and focus!

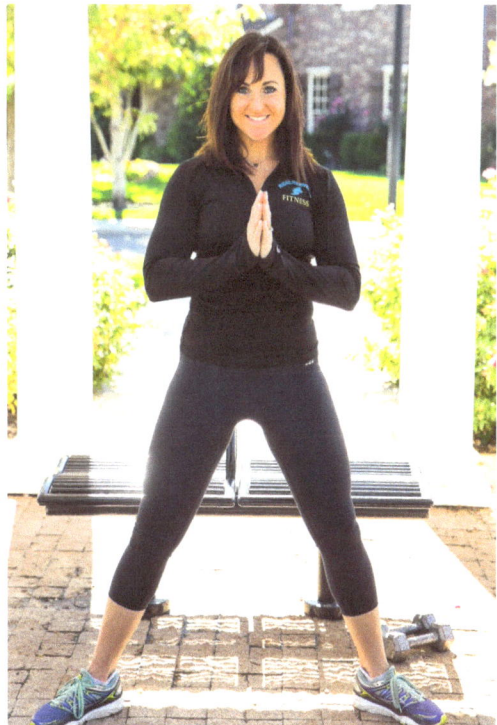

Day 26 Meals: Refer to Chapter 10

Day 26 Movement:
30 Minute Bubble Bath

Day 27 Lifestyle Lesson:
Sweet Feed

While I was growing up, one of my very first jobs was working at my best friend's family-owned feed yard. I would drive a fly spray truck through the yard, mow, and do various odd jobs around the feed yard. Believe it or not, the smell of the yard itself was honestly not that repulsive, but the sickly-sweet smell of the feed mash left a lasting impression. Feed yards strive to get cattle fattened up fast. For profitability, it suits their purpose to feed and finish them in three months instead of three years. To get cattle fattened up quickly, they are fed a concoction of corn, molasses, oats, and wheat called Sweet Feed. To fatten an animal, you don't feed it protein or fat. You don't feed it straight carbohydrates either. The trick is in combining the grainy carbohydrates with sweeteners. The grain/molasses combo produces the perfect layer of fat on the cow for it to be suitable for market.

Pick up that healthy granola bar or cereal box in your pantry and flip it over to the ingredient label:

1)   Maltodextrin (corn derivative)
2)   Oats
3)   Wheat
4)   Molasses, High Fructose Corn Syrup, Cane sugar, Brown Rice Syrup, Agave
5)   Anything ending in -ose (Sucrose, Sucralose, Dextrose, Maltose)

Isn't this ingredient cocktail eerily reminiscent of the Sweet Feed used to fatten up cattle? Refined carbohydrates and sugar will fatten up a woman just like an Angus. Remove these foods from your diet as soon as possible!

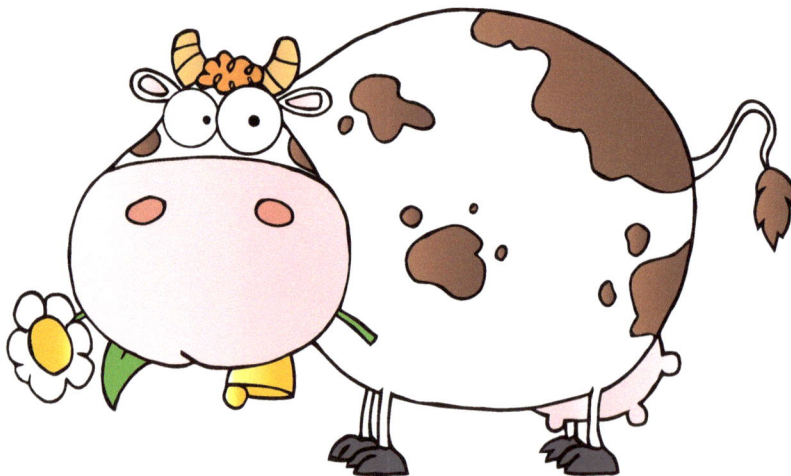

Day 27 Meals: **Refer to Chapter 10**

Day 27 Movement: 10 Minute H.I.I.T. Training
Refer to Chapter 9

Day 28 Lifestyle Lesson:
Sickness Takes Time, So Does Wellness

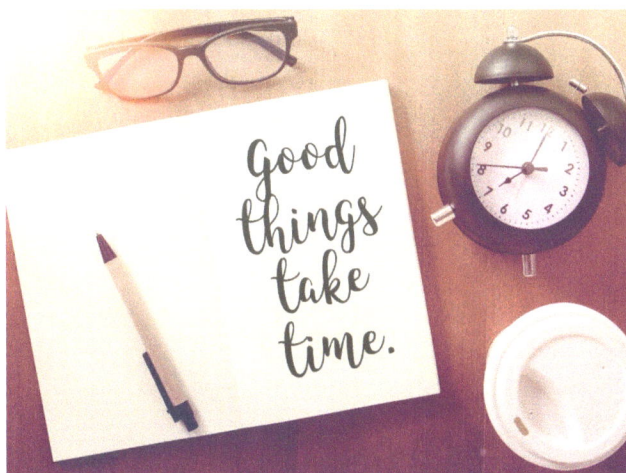

I call this a Health Journey for a reason. There is no "Easy Button" and no fast-forward button. How many years have you been eating fast food, drinking diet sodas, and not moving your body? I am confident it has been more than two months! Maybe even two years? Four years? Joshua Rosenthal, founder of Institute of Integrative Nutrition, coined an invaluable phrase: "The body will heal itself, by itself, given half a chance." This is not to minimize the value of the brilliant physicians in your life, it is to illustrate that if you will remove human error like diet drinks, sedentary lifestyle, processed foods, and sugar from your life, then your body will remember the path to wellness.

Just as interstate highways take time to engineer and construct, your body needs time on this new journey to rebuild itself. Put on your cruise control, roll down the windows, turn up the tunes, and enjoy the ride!

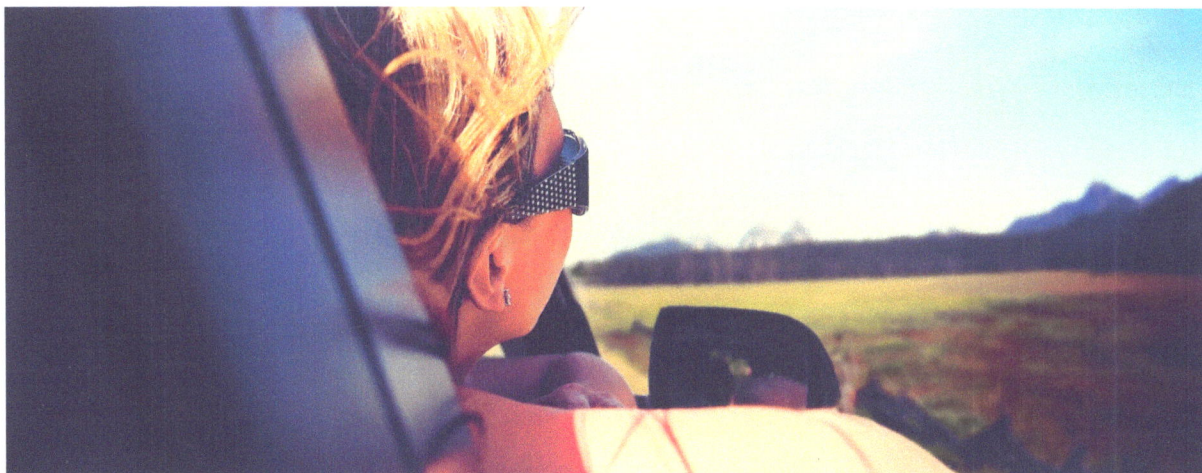

Day 28 Meals: **Refer to Chapter 10**

Day 28 Movement: 15-20 Minute Interval Walk
Refer to Chapter 9

Chapter 8:
"The Road Goes on Forever and the Party Never Ends"

Although the lyrics to Robert Earl Keen's song might not represent our Health Journey, the image of our Highway to Health going off into the sunset does resonate! You are packed and ready for your journey and this party will never end! You have dropped some weight, improved your blood sugar, and changed your mindset regarding food and your emotions. You have the confidence you needed from following this 28-day roadmap. Day by day you checked off items on the packing list:

Air up the tires (saying no to water anorexia): check
Gas up the tank (eliminating the Fattening Five): check
Plan for gas stations along the way (4-7-8 breath): check

Now what?
Now it's time for your Inner Siri to guide you.
1)   Move daily
2)   "Diet" and "Lite" = Red Light!
3)   Live in the Green Zone
4)   Give yourself grace and forgiveness for flat tires
5)   Move from I have to I am!!

Your goal is to continue choosing higher fat, moderate protein, lower carb meals with intentional daily movement. You can start at Day 1 and repeat the weekly meal planner verbatim if you choose! Or you can use the meal planner as a map, and then swap out proteins, veggies, and fats. Use tuna for salmon, raspberries for blueberries, pecans for almonds, or arugula for spinach.

We are blessed to live in the generation of online expertise, and there are some yummy meal plans (roadmap-friendly) just waiting to be discovered by you! I have some favorites that I want to share with you: Kelly Smith's blog The Nourishing Home, Elana Amsterdam's blog, Elana's Pantry, and Maria Emmerich's blog, Maria Mind Body Health.

All of these sources have outstanding recipes and will follow the same style of nutrient combining that we have followed on our Health Journey.

http://thenourishinghome.com/
https://elanaspantry.com/
http://mariamindbodyhealth.com/

We have come to know each other very intimately these past 28 days and I would be honored if you would share your successes with me. Use my contact info at the end of the chapter to **Say Hello!** If you send me your "before" and "after" pictures, I will celebrate your success with you! It can be hard to say goodbye, so I have a list of supports and resources if you need another roadmap:

Nutrition and Fitness extensions:

1)   2-week Bonus meal plan!

http://realresultsfitness.net/index.php?page=book

2)   You can join Real Results! Facebook group for interactive meal prepping and exercise videos $29.99

https://www.facebook.com/groups/847480622086485/?source=create_flow

3) Digital meal and exercise program $49.99

http://realresultsfitness.net/index.php?page=book

4) Skype and Phone sessions $59.99

Jessica@RealResultsFitness.net

Remember, no more Body Naming, Body Blaming, or Body Shaming. Honor your body and she will honor you. May your health journey be as beautiful as you!

Health, Love, and Hope,
Jessica

www.RealResultsFitness.net
Jessica@RealResultsFitness.net

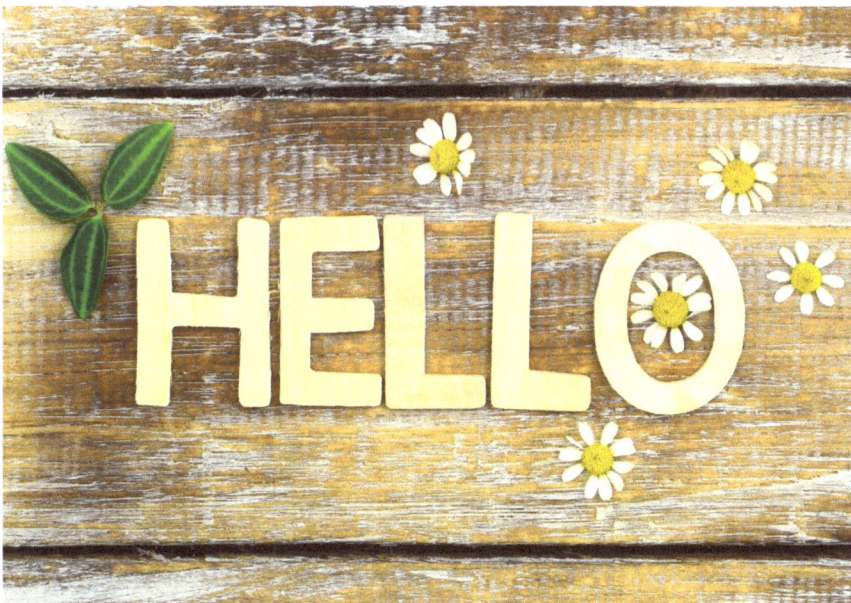

RECIPES

"Diet" = Red Light, remember? This is not a diet plan; this is a food map. If you follow these directions you will create nourishing foods that satisfy not only your body, but your mind and soul as well. This food map is super simple and I have 100% confidence in your ability to follow it.

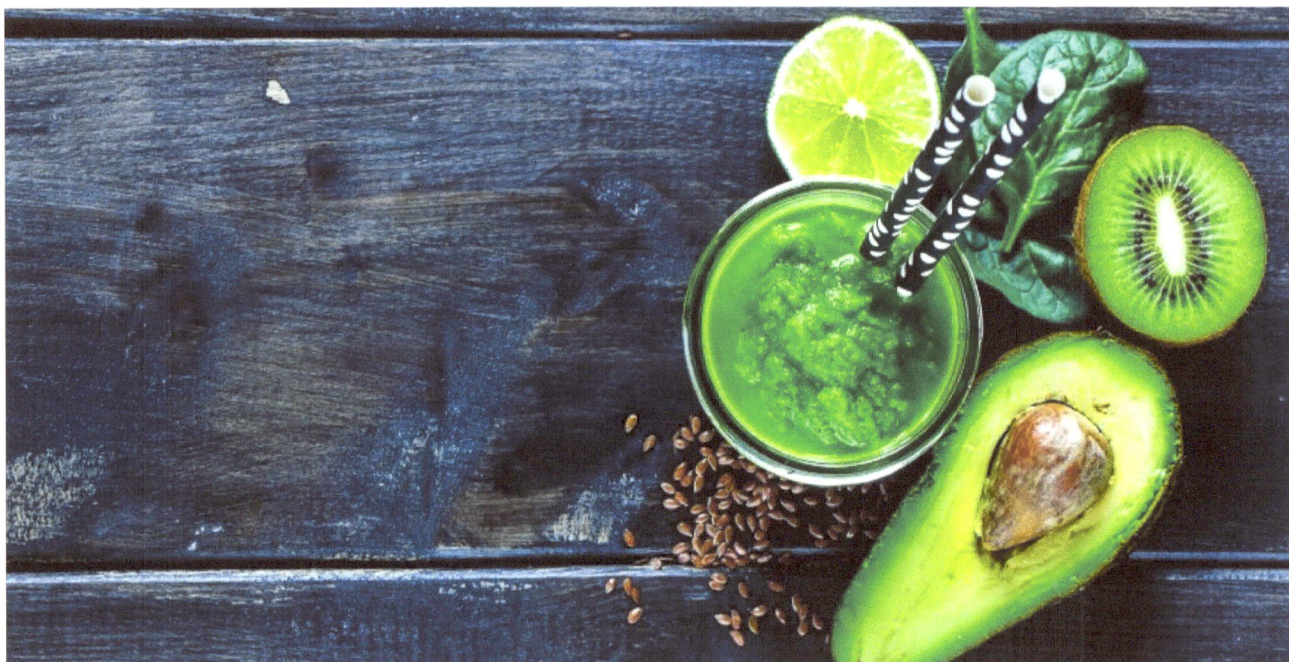

Dosage for the supplements

These supplement suggestions are based on what the average person is missing from his or her daily food choices. If you are working with a practitioner that has already provided you with a list of supplements and dosages specifically for you, then by all means continue! If you are wandering in the dark, then these additions will likely patch some holes on your highway to health.

Probiotic	1 at night
Digestive Enzymes with Betaine HCL	1-2 per meal
Vitamin D3 5000 IU	1 at night
Omega 3 fish oil	1 with dinner

Food for Thought

**ALL dinners include a side salad—use any leftover greens, and a combo of veggies you like. No rules or regulations here! You can have your greens and veggies raw or you can lightly sauté' them with olive oil. If you choose to eat your greens and salad raw and desire a dressing, then choose olive oil and lime/lemon juice. Or find a dressing free from the Fattening Five. Your pantry should now be stocked with hemp hearts, chia seeds, pumpkin seeds, and sunflower seeds-sprinkle them on your salads for good filling fats!

** If you don't have time to cook make a sunrise shake instead!

** If you start into a downward spiral of not making time to cook, fight like you're the third monkey trying to get on Noah's ark! You are building new habits. If it is important to you, you will create time for your meal preparation.

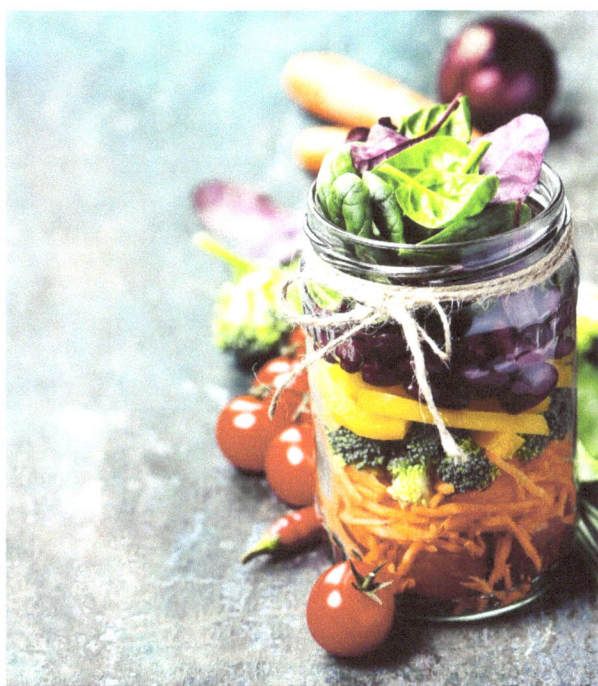

**We are cooking Sunday, Monday, and Tuesday dinners only! The meal prep early in the week balances the crescendo of busy-ness as the week progresses. If you tend to get worn down by Wednesday and Thursday, don't worry! As long as you get the cooking done for Sunday, Monday, and Tuesday you are golden for the other 35 meals that week.

**Entering the Passing Lane sounds exciting, exhilarating even! And it is exhilarating knowing that you don't have to cook on Passing Lane nights!! The word "leftovers" conjures up images of half-eaten, moldy "remains." That mindset is neither appetizing nor an accurate depiction of how we are eating. So even though a rose by any other name would smell as sweet, let's name it something that sounds and smells sweet!

**Scenic Route lunches are designed to give you some freedom and flexibility in your week.

Did you see something at the store you want to try? That's a perfect lunch for today!

Did you see a recipe on Pinterest that meets our guidelines of being Free from the Fattening Five? Bring it on!

I have also included a few bonus recipes that you can pull from to experiment with on your Scenic Route lunches.

Remember, the goal is to lower cortisol and stress response, so if you feel anxiety rising by having to plan something to eat, just eat what is left from the week or make a shake. Be cool, calm, and collected—the goal is to enjoy the food not stress over it.

**Treats versus Cheats

Treats = rewards, excitement, expectation
Cheats = guilt, shame, remorse

Please do not cheat on yourself with food. Food is an inanimate object, void of any emotion or attachment, so it can't even cheat back with you! If there are foods that you love and miss then budget to have them as a treat. Plan for it; be intentional—not impulsive—so that you enjoy the treat and spare yourself the self-deprecating emotions of guilt, shame, and remorse.

Even your treats need to be Free from the Fattening Five.
 If your treats start making daily appearances, they are no longer treats—they have become a habit and need to be removed.

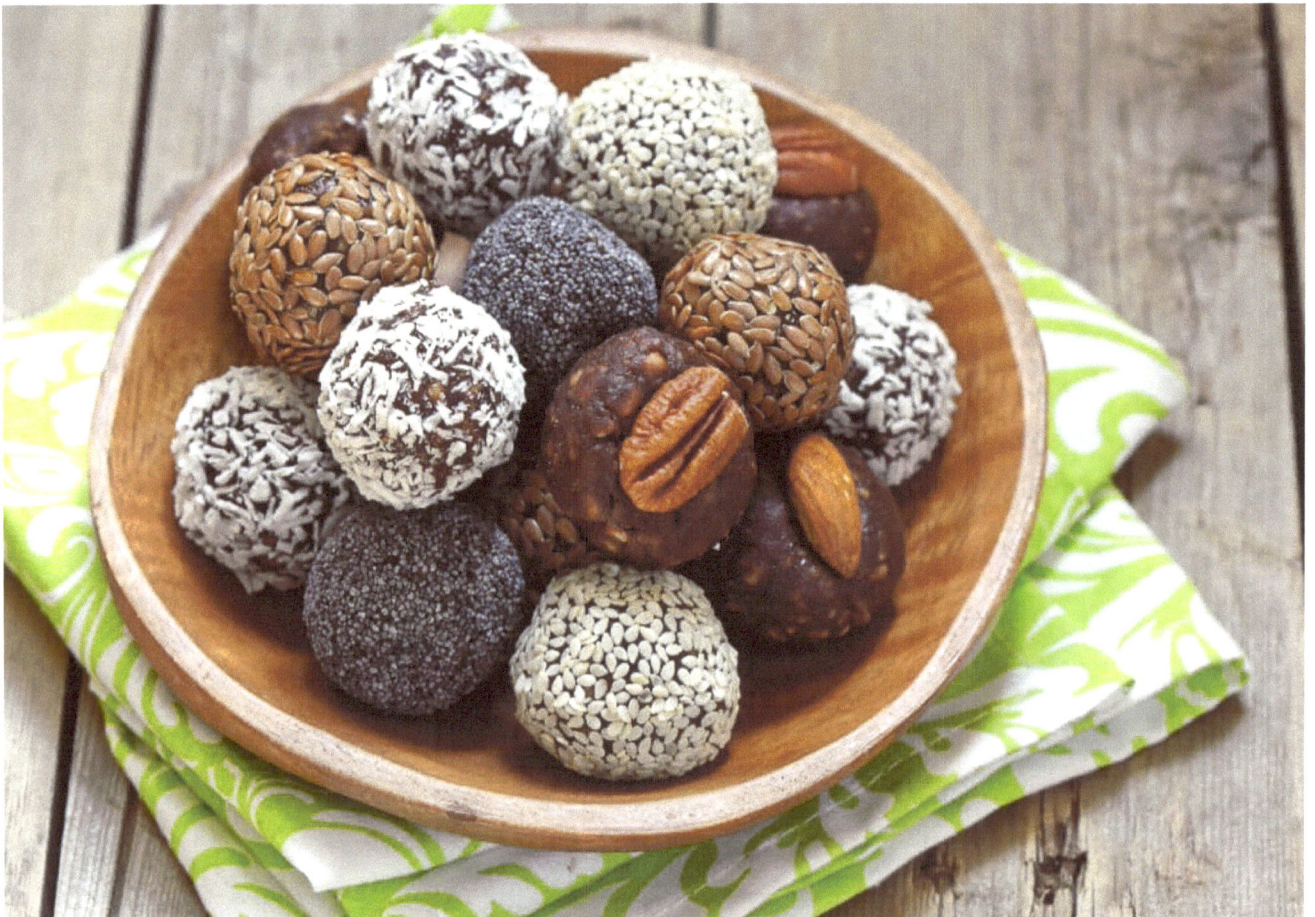

SutterBites

BREAKFASTS

BULLETPROOF COFFEE
A delicious and creamy coffee that packs a powerful nutritional punch!
1 Serving; Prep time: 5 minutes

- 1 cup of brewed coffee or chai tea
- 1 tsp. coconut oil (or more, I usually put in 1 Or you can use MCT oil
- 1 organic unsalted butter
- ½ vanilla
- a few drops of stevia extract (optional)
- a few sprinkles of cinnamon

Put all ingredients in a blender or food processor. Mix on high speed for 20 seconds until frothy.

CHOCOLATE COVERED CHERRY SMOOTHIE

2 servings; Prep 5 minutes
Blend all ingredients and drink immediately. Can be any meal replacement or a pre-post workout boost.

- 2 cups pitted cherries
- 1 cup plain unsweetened kefir or yogurt
- ½ cup unsweetened almond or coconut milk
- 2 scoops clean chocolate protein powder (Free from the Fattening 5)
- 1 vanilla extract
- 1-2 drops stevia if needed
- 1 dark chocolate (60% or more) baking cocoa (optional)
- Ice cubes to thicken, if desired

***This is two servings. Drink one serving and store the remainder in a freezer stable container to be breakfast on Saturday. Transfer container from freezer to refrigerator Friday afternoon. **

GOOD MORNING BURRITO

2 servings (1 as a snack) Prep 10 minutes, Cook 5 minutes

- 3 whole eggs
- 1-2 cup chopped veggies of choice (mushrooms, spinach, bell peppers, onions, broccoli—have fun with it!)
- ½ cup precooked chicken or deli chicken or bacon
- 3 Tbsp. salsa or pico de gallo
- 4-5 slices avocado
- 1 cabbage leaf, romaine leaf, or sprouted tortilla
- Spray skillet with coconut cooking spray. Heat pan to medium and sauté veggies for 3-4 minutes. Add egg mixture and stir continuously. Serve in wrapper or serve in a bowl and eat with a fork!

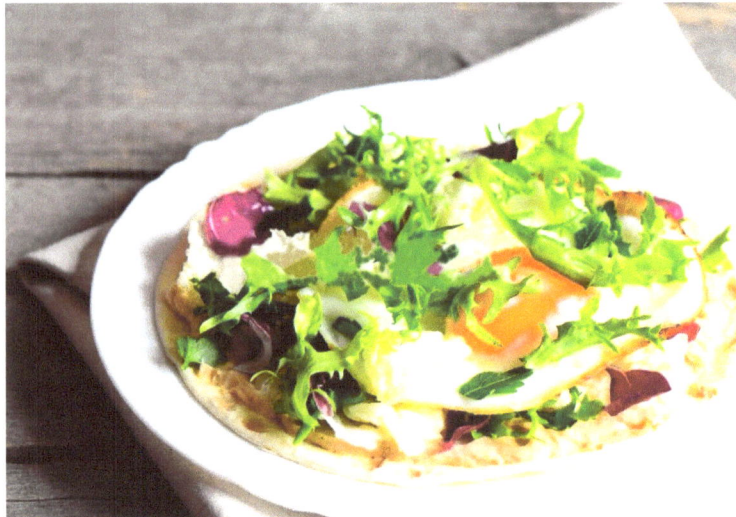

JESSICA MCMUFFIN

24 McMuffins; Prep time: 20 minutes; Bake time: 20-25 minutes
- 2-3 McMuffins is a serving
- 10 eggs
- Celtic sea salt and pepper to taste
- 1 garlic salt
- ½ onion
- 10oz cooked meat or deli meat (shredded chicken, sausage, bacon, ground beef, ham—your call!)
- 1 red bell pepper
- 2-3 cups fresh spinach
- ¾ cup organic cheese
- 2 Tbsp. chia seeds (optional)

Preheat oven to 350 degrees and grease 2 (12 count) muffin tins. Whisk eggs with seasonings. Chop onion and bell pepper and mix into egg mixture. Next, tear off and discard the spinach stems and add spinach leaves to the eggs. Add remaining ingredients and mix well. Use a 1/3 measuring cup to fill each tin. Bake for 20-25 minutes until eggs are set. These can be frozen for a quick on the go breakfast or lunch! Kept well in fridge for one week.

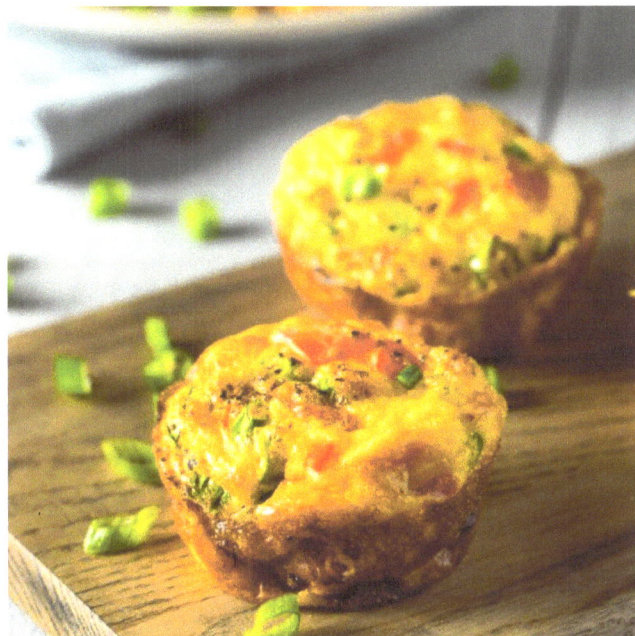

**If you make 24 McMuffins then you have week 2 and week 4 done! Keep 12 McMuffins in the fridge for week 1 and freeze the other 12 to pull out the Saturday before week 4.

MEXICAN EGG OMELET

2 servings (1 as a snack); Prep 5 minutes, Cook 10 minutes

- 2 tsp. olive oil
- 1 small jalapeno, thinly sliced and seeded (if desired), stem discarded
- ½ cup premade pico de gallo
- 1 tsp. minced garlic
- salt and pepper
- 4 eggs
- half an avocado, peeled, pitted and diced
- chopped fresh cilantro, dried will work
- crumbled organic cheese

DIRECTIONS:

Heat oil in a medium sauté pan over medium heat. Add jalapeno, garlic, and pico and sauté for 3-4 minutes, stirring occasionally. Season to taste with a pinch of salt and pepper. Then transfer the mixture to a separate plate.

Return pan to the stove, and reduce heat to medium. Spray pan with coconut spray or add a touch more olive oil if needed. Add the whisked eggs and cook for 2-3 minutes until the eggs are set and the bottom of the egg is golden. Remove from heat. Add the Pico mixture, diced avocado, cilantro and cheese to the egg, and fold over to form the omelet. Serve warm, garnished with extra cilantro and cheese if desired. **Tip** Buy block cheese, organic if feasible. Grate the cheese yourself to avoid preservatives and extra processing.

MORNING LIVER LOVER

- 16oz water
- 1 Tbsp. lemon juice
- 1 tsp. ACV

Drink first thing-before brushing teeth each morning.

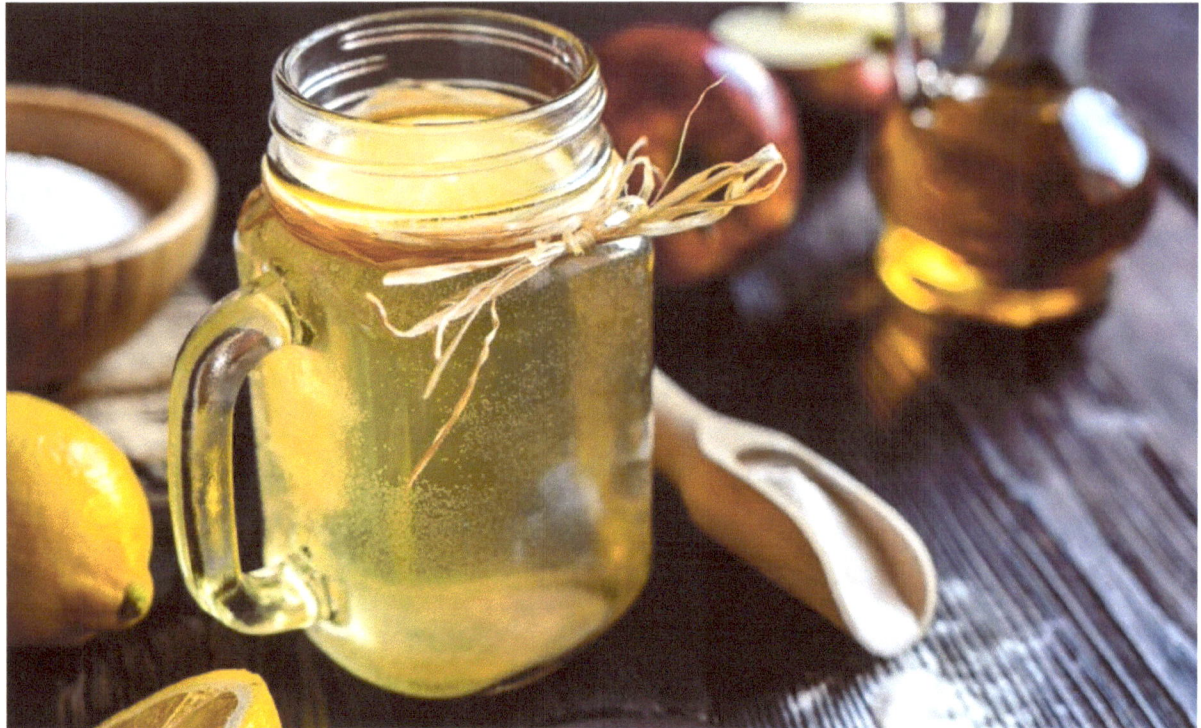

PUMPKIN SPICE LATTE
2 servings; Prep time: 5 minutes

- 1 cup vanilla unsweet coconut or almond milk
- ½ cup plain pumpkin purée filling
- 1 ½ scoops vanilla whey protein (must be free from the Fattening 5)
- 1 tbsp. vanilla extract
- 1-2 drops stevia
- 1-2 tsp. pumpkin pie spice (can just use cinnamon if desired)
- 10 oz strong brewed coffee

Blend all ingredients and drink immediately. Can be any meal replacement or a pre-or post-workout boost. If you are prepping this the night before, then put all ingredients in the blender and refrigerate-—don't freeze,—overnight.   Simply blend in the morning.

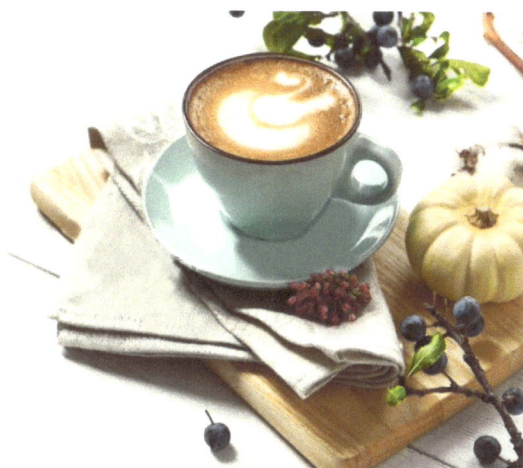

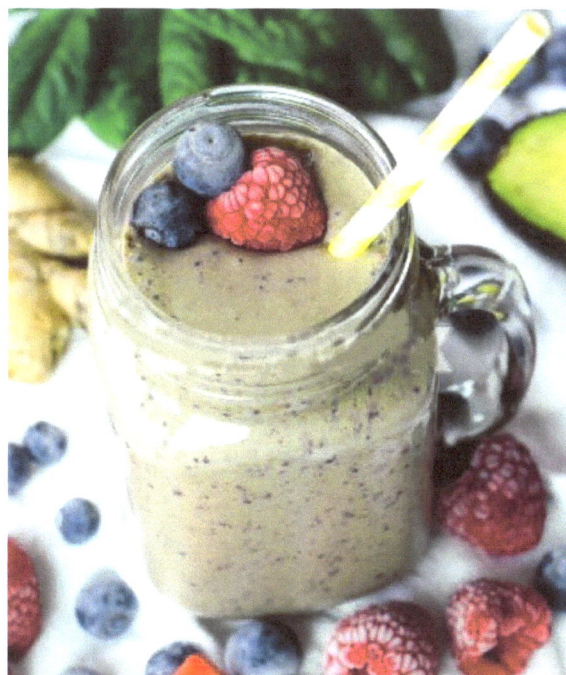

SUNRISE SHAKE
1 serving; Prep 5 minutes

- 1 scoop vanilla whey protein
- 3 cups fresh spinach, stems removed
- ½ cup blueberries
- 2 Tbsp. almond butter
- ¾ cup vanilla unsweetened coconut or almond milk
- 2 cups ice

Blend all ingredients and drink immediately. Can be any meal replacement or a pre-or post-workout boost. If you are prepping this the night before, then put all ingredients in the blender and refrigerate—don't freeze—overnight. Simply blend in the morning.

LUNCHES

BERRY COLORFUL SALAD
1 servings; Prep 10 minutes

- 4 oz leftover chicken, turkey, ham or use nitrate free deli meat
- 1 loose cup of mixed berries: blueberries, raspberries, blackberries, strawberries
- ¼ cup hemp hearts
- 3 cups leafy greens or spring mix
- 2 Tbsp. balsamic vinegar or lime juice

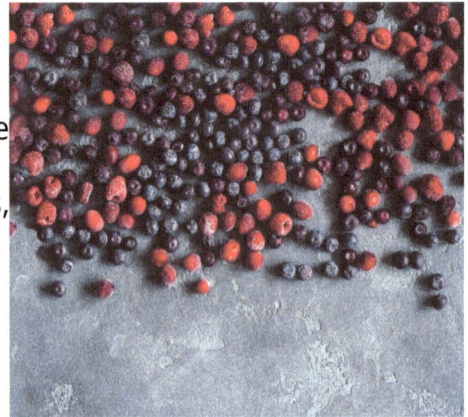

Everything in a bowl, smile while you smack!

LETTUCE WRAPS

For week 3, wrap leftover Melt in Your Mouth chicken, Tuna Patty with Personality, and Mexican chicken in green leafy lettuce or cabbage leaves. You can stuff the meat in a bell pepper if preferred. Add cheese if desired.
For week 4, wrap leftover BBQ chicken and Orange chicken in green leafy lettuce or cabbage wraps. You can stuff the meat in a bell pepper if preferred. Add cheese if desired.

HAMWICH

1 serving; Prep 5 minutes, Cook 5 minutes of frying if desired

- 2 thick slices of nitrate free ham such as Beeler's or Pederson's
- 1 (2oz.) thick slice of favorite cheese
- 2 Tbsp. Avocado or olive oil mayo
- 1/8 tsp. each Seasonings such as dill, cilantro, salt, pepper, and crushed red pepper
- Thin sliced pickles—-must be free of dyes and additives.

Mix 2 Tbsp. of mayo with seasonings to taste. Trim the casing layer off and discard. If you are at home you can brown both sides of the ham in a skillet for a treat! For on the go, simply layer ham then mayo, then pickle then cheese then last piece of ham. Or for a change you can roll the ham and cheese up in a thin sliced cucumber! I usually roll the cheese inside of the ham and eat it as a roll.

NUTTY BUT NICE SALAD
1 serving; Prep 10 minutes

- 4 oz. leftover chicken, beef, or use nitrate-free deli meat
- 3 cups leafy greens or spring mix
- 1/2 cup nuts and shredded unsweet coconut flakes
- 2 Tbsp. sunflower seeds
- ½ avocado, or 1/3 cup guacamole
- 2 Tbsp. balsamic vinegar or lime juice

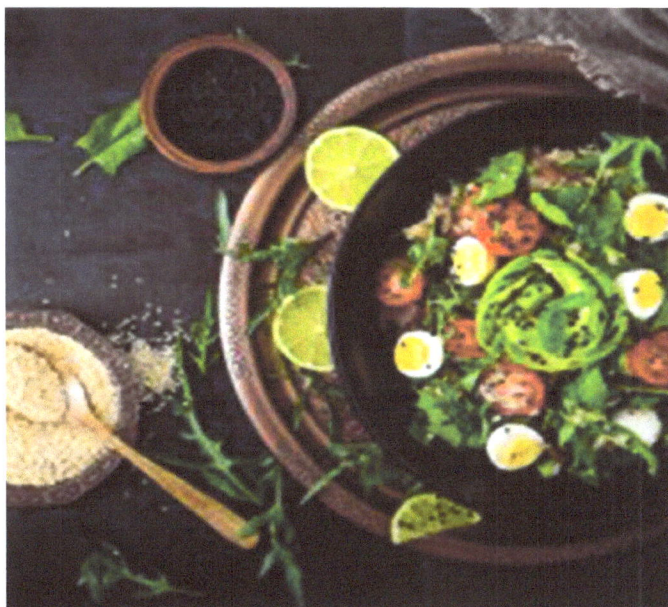

SHREDDED ROAST BEEF IN BELL PEPPERS
1 Serving; Prep time: 5 minutes, Bake time: 10 minutes

- 4 oz. Leftover roast (or deli meat nitrate free)
- 1 bell pepper
- ¼ cup cheese
- Seasonings as desired: BBQ sauce, Mexican seasonings, or just salt and pepper.

Wash the bell pepper and chop the top off. Core the inside, leaving the solid bell pepper to be used as a cup. Stuff the meat and cheese in the bell pepper cup. This can be eaten cold, or you can heat it in the oven at 350 degrees for 10 minutes.

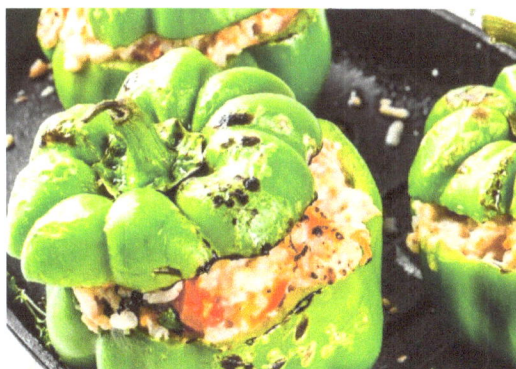

SUNDAY HAM
4 servings; Prep time: 5 minutes, Bake time: 10 minutes

- 1-lb natural precooked Ham (I like the Beeler's ham)
- 2 Tbsp. maple syrup
- 1 Tbsp. balsamic vinegar
- Seasonings to taste: minced garlic, salt, pepper, cayenne

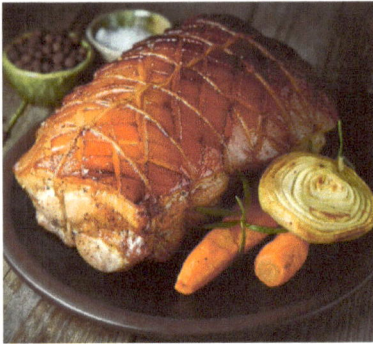

Unwrap the ham from the plastic and discard the juice and plastic. Place the ham with casings facing up in a small baking dish and cover with foil. Heat at 350 degrees until warm. Meanwhile bring the liquids and seasonings to a low rolling boil in a small pan. Remove the ham from the oven and use a knife to create 8 slices. Save 4 slices for the Hamwich later in the week. Trim the casings off the slices and discard. Drizzle 2 tsp. of sauce onto the ham and serve with a salad or veggie mix.

SUNDAY ROAST (CROCKPOT)
4 servings; Prep time: 10 minutes, Cook time: 6-8 hours

- 2 lbs. Boneless Chuck Roast
- ½ cup paleo mayo
- 2 Tbsp. olive oil
- 2 Tbsp. minced garlic
- Salt, pepper

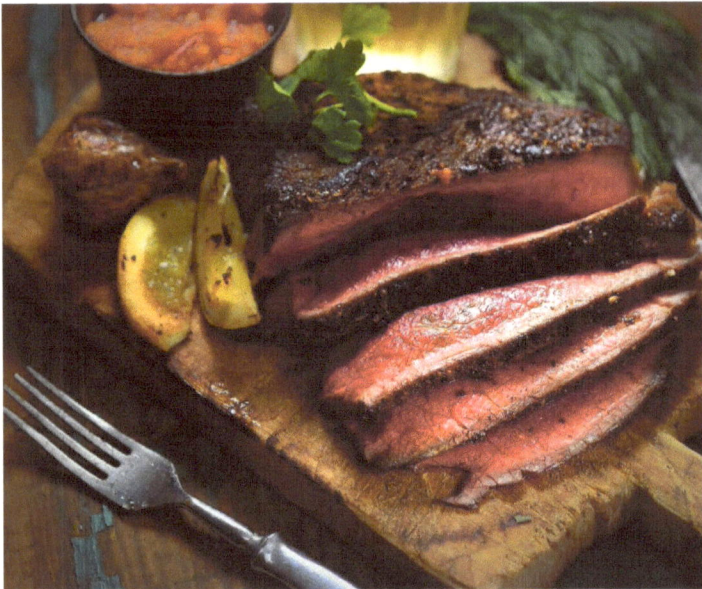

Brown the roast on all sides in a skillet. While browning the roast pour olive oil inside crockpot and turn on low heat. Transfer the browned roast to the crockpot. Toss and turn the roast a few times to be sure that it is covered in the oil. Sprinkle the seasoning and garlic on roast. Pour the mayo over the roast and spread with a spoon. Cover and cook on low for 6-8 hours.

DINNERS

2 INGREDIENT ITALIAN CHICKEN
4 servings; Prep 10 minutes, Cook 10 minutes

- 4 Boneless skinless chicken breasts
- 1 cup organic Italian herb spaghetti sauce or marinade

You can choose any type of spaghetti sauce; I love the 4 cheese Organics brand. Check label to be free of the Fattening 5.

If you have time, marinate in sauce the night before. Cut chicken into small cubes. Spray skillet with nonstick spray (preferably coconut spray). Add chicken to heated skillet and stir occasionally until it is cooked through (no pink in the middle). Sauté sliced zucchini in same pan if desired. Can top with dried or fresh cilantro and basil. Serve with 2 cups of arugula/spinach or half and half greens.

2 INGREDIENT SALMON BOATS
4 servings; Prep 10 minutes, Cook 30 minutes

- 4 frozen or fresh salmon fillets (6oz. each)
- ½ cup olive oil or primal mayo (sir Kensington)
- Optional but yummy-1 tsp. each: Celtic sea salt, garlic salt, onion salt, (basil and cilantro if desired)

Preheat oven to 350 degrees. Place salmon fillets in individual foil boats (large enough to wrap and close) Place all boats on a cookie sheet. Mix the mayo and seasonings. Put 2 Tbsp. mix on each fillet. Tightly wrap up the foil without touching the fillet. Bake for 20 minutes. Open foil boats and bake additional 10 minutes or until fillets flake with a fork.

BBQ CHICKEN LETTUCE WRAPS (CROCKPOT)
4 servings; Prep 10 minutes, Cook 6-8 hours or high 4 hours

- 4 chicken breasts fresh or thawed (6oz. each)
- 1 cup clean BBQ low in sugar (Fattening 5 Free)
- 1 red onion sliced
- 2 carrots grated
- 8 or more leaves of green leafy lettuce

Place chicken breasts in crockpot and cover with the clean BBQ sauce. Mix chicken so BBQ sauce fully coats the chicken breasts. Be sure the chicken breasts are lying flat at the bottom of the crockpot so they cook evenly. Top with onions and carrots. Turn the crockpot on high for 4 hours or low for 6-8 hours. Shred the chicken in the crockpot with two forks. Spoon the carrots, onions, and chicken into the lettuce wraps.

BEEF FAJITAS
4 servings; Prep 10 minutes, marinate 30 minutes, Cook 10 minutes

- 1.5lbs flank steak or precut fajita meat (don't buy seasoned meat unless the seasonings are void of the Fattening 5)
- 2 red, yellow or green bell peppers
- 1 white or yellow onion
- 5 thin asparagus spears
- 1 cup premade pico de gallo or salsa
- 1 package wholly guacamole or sliced avocado
- 1 lime or 2-3 Tbsp. lime juice
- 1 package clean fajita seasoning mix or use these spices to taste: cayenne, garlic, onion, chili powder
- Sprouted tortillas, cabbage leaf, or big green leafy lettuce

Slice meat into strips. Rough chop or slice the veggies. Season meat, add lime juice and let marinate overnight or 30 minutes. Spray skillet with coconut cooking spray and heat to medium. Add marinated meat and stir till only slightly pink in middle. Add all veggies and continue cooking for another 2-4 minutes. Remove from heat. Fill a tortilla or lettuce leaf with meat mixture, add Pico and guacamole.

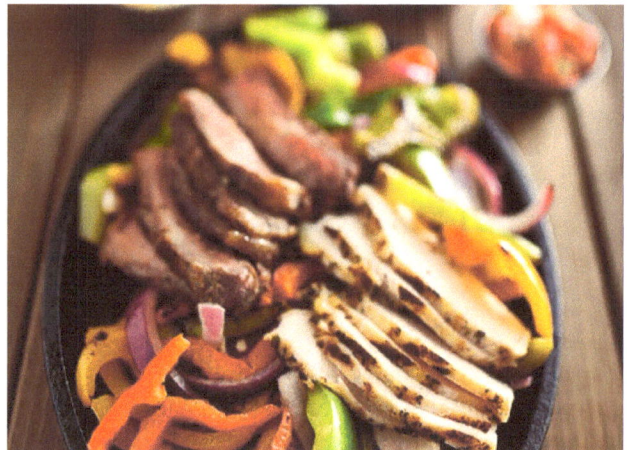

MEAT ONLY MEATLOAF
4 servings, Prep 5 minutes, Cook 45 minutes

- 2lbs ground beef
- 1 tsp.Celtic sea salt
- 2 tsp. ground black pepper
- ½ to 1 package chipotle ranch seasoning mix (Fattening 5 Free)
- 1 cup shredded gouda or Colby cheese
- ½ cup oat flour
- 2 eggs mixed
- ¼ cup pure maple syrup

Mix the seasonings and flour together in medium bowl. Add the meat and mix well. Add the cheese and maple syrup and mix well. Finally add the eggs. Bake in 13x9 dish at 350 degrees for 40-50 minutes (check often as ovens are variable!).

MELT IN YOUR MOUTH CHICKEN (CROCKPOT)
4 servings; Prep 10 minutes, Cook 6-8 hours on low or 4 hours on high

- 4 chicken breasts 6 oz. each
- 1 cup paleo mayo
- ½ cup freshly grated parmesan or gouda cheese
- 1 tsp. Celtic sea salt
- ½ tsp. black pepper
- ½ package of ranch seasoning (free from Fattening 5)
- 2 tsp. minced garlic
- 3 pieces cooked bacon, crumbled

Mix everything but chicken in glass bowl. Place chicken flat and evenly in slow cooker and top with the mayo mixture. Cook on low for 6-8 hours. Add more mayo if it appears to be dry. Bake bacon at 350 degrees for 20 minutes and crumble on top of chicken before serving.

MEXICAN CHICKEN
4 servings; Prep 10 minutes, Cook 45 minutes

- 4 thawed or fresh chicken breasts (6oz. each)
- 1 package taco seasoning (free from the Fattening 5)
- 1 cup salsa or pico de gallo premade
- ¼ cup grated cheese
- 1 egg cooked over easy for each chicken breast (during the 5-minute cheese melt)
- 2-3 slices of avocado per serving
- 3 pieces cooked bacon, crumbled

Thaw breasts overnight and pat dry. If you try to marinate with the mix the remaining juices will get rinsed away. Spray your baking dish with coconut oil. Preheat oven to 350 degrees. Roll chicken in the taco seasoning and place in dish. Top with salsa. Bake covered at 350 degrees for 40-45 minutes. Take pan out and sprinkle cheese on top. Bake uncovered another 5 minutes. Top with the over-easy egg and slice of avocado.

ORANGE CHICKEN (CROCKPOT)
4 servings; Prep time: 10 minutes; Cook time: 6-8 hours + 20 minutes to thicken the sauce

- 2lb chicken breasts cubed
- ½ cup coconut amino sauce (soy sauce substitute can be found in the gluten free section)
- ¼ - ½ cup raw honey
- ½ cup orange juice
- ¼ cup sesame oil
- 1 Tbsp. minced garlic
- 1/2 tsp. ground ginger
- 3/4 tsp. sea salt
- 1/2 tsp. cayenne
- 1/4 tsp. black pepper

Put chicken flat and evenly in crockpot. Mix all ingredients together and pour over chicken to coat. Cook for 6-8 hours on low. Pour sauce into small sauce pan and simmer for 20 min to reduce and thicken. Pour back in crockpot over chicken. Garnish with sesame seeds if desired.

PORTABELLA CHEESEBURGER
4 servings; Prep 10 minutes, Cook 15 minutes

- 2.5 lbs ground beef
- 4-6 portabella mushrooms
- 1-2 Tbsp. olive oil
- 2-3 tsp. cumin
- 1/2 tsp. cayenne
- 1 tsp. ground ginger
- Salt, pepper, garlic to taste
- 2 Tbsp. maple syrup
- Toppings:
- 1/3 cup guacamole or ½ avocado
- Sautéed or fresh onions, tomatoes, and lettuce as desired
- Green chilis for topping if desired

While the grill or skillet is heating, mix all the seasonings and syrup in glass bowl. Add the meat and mix thoroughly. Use hands to roll into balls. Flatten into patties on a plate. Prep a grill or skillet with coconut oil and cook patties till no pink is visible, flipping as necessary. When burgers are almost finished, brush portabella cap with oil and grill till brown, about 3 minutes. Or you can broil in the oven at 500 degrees for 1 minute.

Top with guacamole or avocado, sautéed or fresh onions, lettuce and tomatoes. Green chilis make a nice treat!

Substitute romaine lettuce leaf if opposed to mushrooms. Or eat with a fork!

ROASTED RANCH CHICKEN
4 servings; Prep 10 minutes, Cook 25 minutes

- 4 thawed or fresh chicken breasts (6 oz. each)
- 1 package clean ranch or chipotle ranch mix (Fattening 5 Free)
- 2 Tbsp. olive oil
- 1 cup chicken broth
- 1 Tbsp. balsamic vinegar
- ½ Tbsp. minced garlic
- 3 green onions chopped
- 1 cup frozen green beans or Brussels sprouts

Thaw breasts overnight and pat dry. If you try to marinate with the mix, the remaining juices will get rinsed away. Brush chicken breasts with oil then sprinkle thoroughly with ranch mix. Heat large skillet to medium and 1 Tbsp. olive oil. Add seasoned chicken and cook 3 minutes per side. Remove chicken from skillet and place in 13x9 baking pan. Bake 15-20 minutes or until no longer pink.

Meanwhile add garlic, green onions, and green beans or Brussels sprouts to the hot skillet (leave the oil and bits of chicken) Sauté 3-5 minutes. Reduce heat to low, add broth and simmer 5 minutes. Add balsamic vinegar and simmer another minute while removing chicken from oven. Add salt and pepper to taste. Serve sauce over chicken

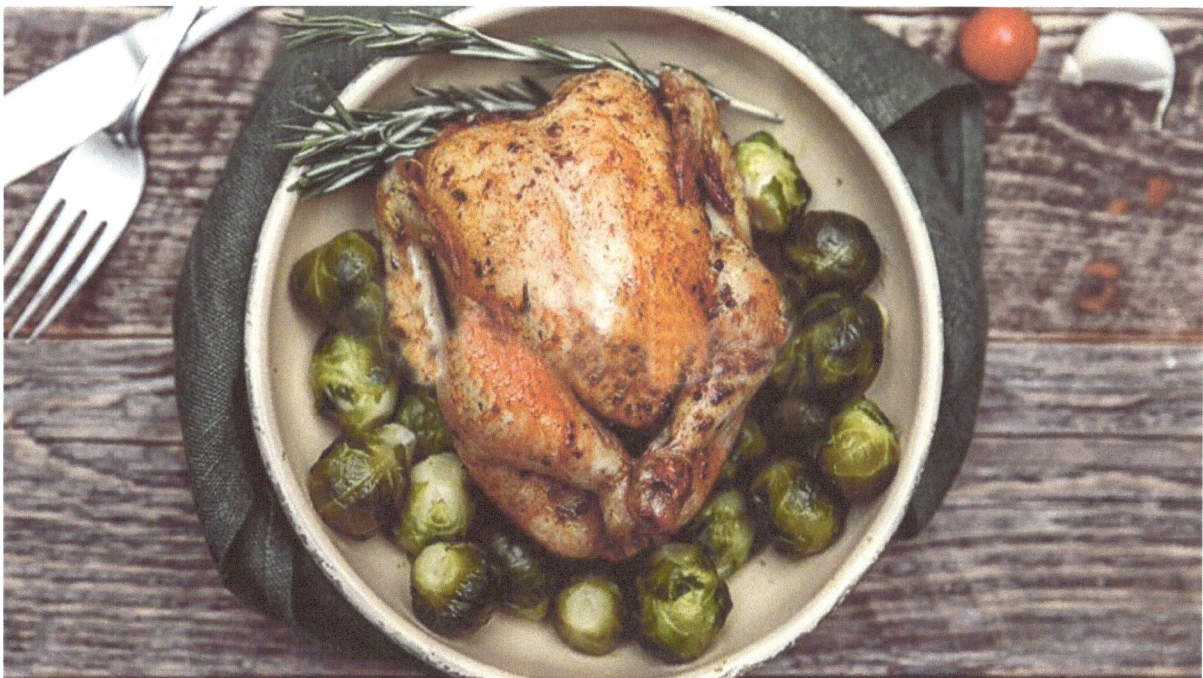

SPICY SALMON
4 servings; Prep 45 minutes, Cook 10 minutes

- 4 frozen or fresh salmon fillets (6 oz. each)
- 1 Tbsp. extra virgin olive oil
- 4 Tbsp. lime juice
- 1 tsp. each: sea salt, black pepper, garlic, onion
- ½ tsp. each: cayenne pepper, cinnamon
- Topping:
- 1 container premade Pico de Gallo
- 1 avocado sliced

Mix marinade in large glass bowl, add fish and coat thoroughly. Marinade overnight or 30 minutes at least. Spray skillet with nonstick spray (preferably coconut spray). Add salmon to heated skillet and cook for 5 minutes, turn fillets and cook another 4-5 minutes until fish flakes easily. Transfer salmon to plate and top with 1/3 cup of salsa and 3 slices avocado. Serve with 2 cups of arugula/spinach or half and half greens.

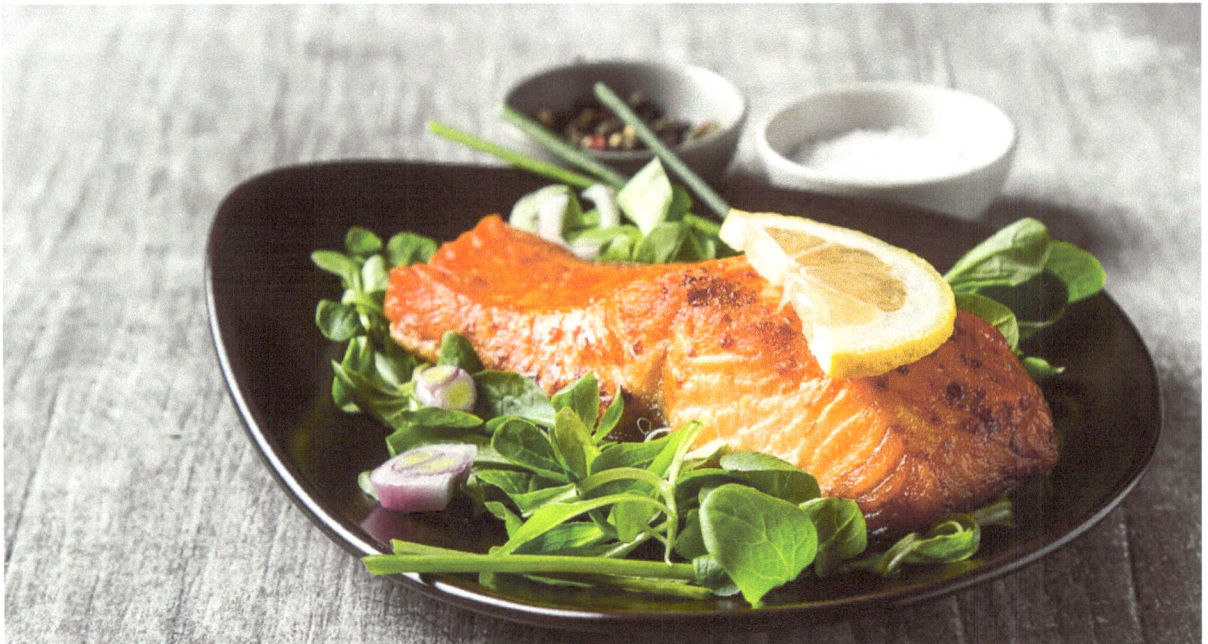

TUNA PATTIES WITH PERSONALITY
4 servings; Prep 10 minutes, Cook 25 minutes

- 3, 6-oz. cans tuna in spring water; drained
- 1 egg beaten
- 8 slices bacon
- 1 white or yellow onion
- ½ Tbsp. minced or dried garlic
- 1 Tbsp. honey or maple syrup
- 1 tsp. each: cumin, ginger, Celtic sea salt, pepper

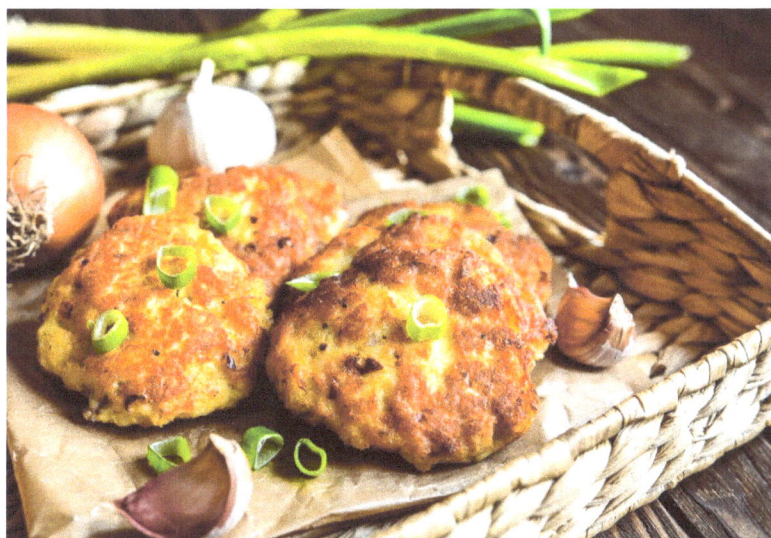

Drain the tuna and put into glass bowl. Lay bacon flat in skillet on medium-high. While bacon cooks chop the onion. Add the onion and garlic to the cooking bacon. Meanwhile beat the egg and mix thoroughly into the tuna. Remove the bacon from the pan and crumble into a small dish. Add the maple syrup and spices to the bacon while hot. Add the bacon mixture to the tuna mixture and shape into 4 balls. Flatten and press into the skillet. (If there is a lot of grease, then drain all but 1 Tbsp. of the bacon grease.) Brown the tuna for 2-3 minutes on each side on medium high heat. Serve with fresh or steamed veggies.

SNACKS

BLISS SNACK BARS
18 servings: Prep time: 10 minutes, Bake time: 15 minutes

- 1 ½ cup unsweetened shredded coconut
- 1 cup chopped walnuts, pecans, or almonds (or a mix of all 3!)
- 2/3 cup chia seeds
- 1/2 cup pumpkin seeds
- 1/2 cup sunflower seeds
- 1/2 cup ground flax seed
- 1/2 cup dark chocolate chips
- 1 tsp. sea salt
- 1/2 cup maple syrup
- 1/2 cup almond butter

1. Preheat oven to 350ºF. Line a square 8×8 pan with parchment paper and lightly oil with coconut oil.

2. Mix all ingredients (except syrup and almond butter) in a large mixing bowl.

3. Add syrup and almond butter into the mixing bowl and stir until all ingredients are evenly distributed.

4. Transfer mix into the pan and press down firmly.

5. Bake in the oven for 15 minutes.

6. Remove from oven and let cool completely (place pan in the freezer to speed the cooling process). Once cool, lift parchment paper out of the tin and slice into 10 bars with a sharp knife.

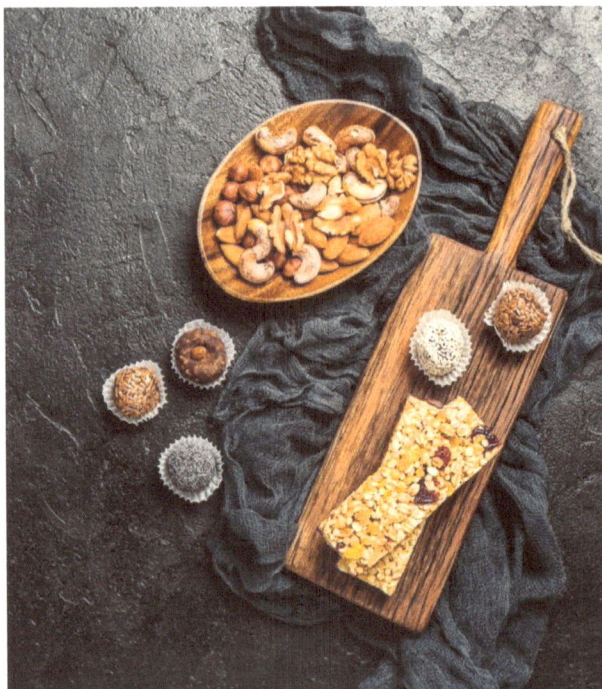

CHOCOLATE CHIP COOKIE DOUGH
24 balls; Serving 3 balls; Prep time 10 minutes

- 1 cup all-natural peanut butter, creamy or crunchy (I use almond butter)
- 1 cup oat flour (see Notes to find out how to make your own)
- 2 tsp. vanilla extract
- 1/3 cup honey or maple syrup
- 3 scoops vanilla protein powder
- ½ cup dark chocolate chips

1. Measure all ingredients into a large bowl. Use a large spoon or spatula to thoroughly combine the ingredients until the mixture forms a thick dough. Make sure there aren't any dry bits left in the bottom of the bowl.

2. Using a 1-tablespoon-sized cookie scoop, portion out the mixture and roll into 24 balls. Place finished balls on a large plate. You can flatten them into cookie shapes now or eat them as balls.

3. Refrigerate balls until set, about 45 minutes and then transfer to an airtight container (it's okay to stack them).

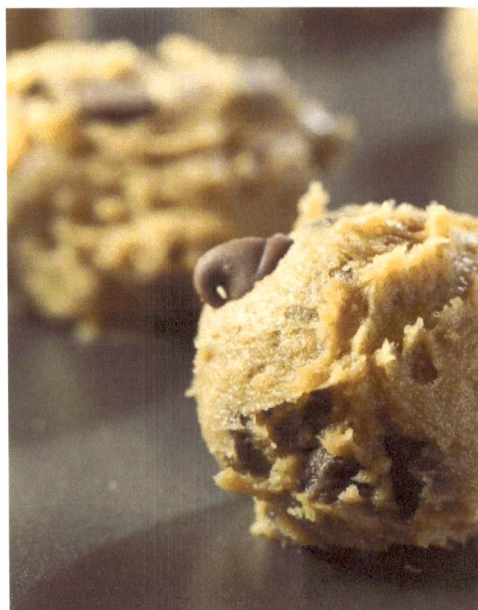

4. Freeze

RECIPE NOTES:

• To make your own oat flour, place rolled oats in a blender or food processor and pulse until oats completely break down and form a fine flour. Store any leftover flour in an airtight container in the refrigerator.

• Feel free to experiment with other kinds of nut butter, other flavors of protein powder, and other mix-ins (such as seeds, chopped nuts, or coconut flakes). If your mixture becomes too dry, add more peanut butter or honey one tablespoon at a time until mixture is once again malleable.

JESSICA'S JAZZY TRAIL MIX
10 servings; Prep time 5 minutes, bake time 0-15 minutes depending on method.

- Serving is ½ cup
- 5 cups nut combination (pecans, walnuts, macadamias, cashews, almonds
- 2 cups shredded unsweet coconut flakes
- 1 cup dark chocolate chunks (my favorite thing to do is to buy quality bars like Theo or Alter Eco and break those up into chunks—it's cheaper that way as well!)
- ½ cup hemp hearts
- 1 tsp.Celtic sea salt

Fast route: Pour all of the ingredients into a huge bowl, cover with a lid and shake to mix. Portion the mix into individual snack size baggies.

Tastier Route: Lay the nuts flat on baking dish and toast at 400 degrees for 10 minutes. Transfer the nuts to a large bowl and pour the coconut flakes onto the baking dish. Toast the coconut flakes for 2-3 minutes watching the entire time to avoid burnt coconut! Transfer the coconut flakes and remaining ingredients to the large bowl. If you want the chocolate to melt over the nuts then immediately mix all ingredients. Shake well and portion into snack size baggies.

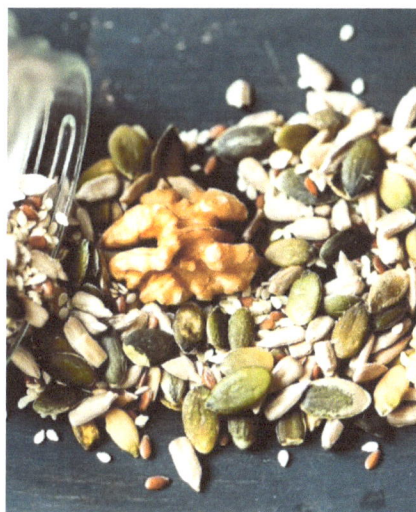

PALEO SOUTHERN BISCUITS
Author: Reprinted with permission from Everyday Grain-Free Baking
Serves: 16 biscuits; Prep time: 10 minutes, bake time 15 minutes

- 5 cups blanched almond flour
- 1 tsp. baking soda
- 1/2 tsp. sea salt
- 6 Tbsp. unsalted butter (or coconut oil), melted
- 4 Tbsp. honey
- 4 Tbsp. coconut milk or almond milk
- 4 large eggs
- ½ teaspoon apple cider vinegar
- 3-4 tablespoons cinnamon (Jessica addition)

1. Preheat oven to 350°F. Line a baking sheet with parchment paper; set aside.
2. In a small bowl, combine almond flour, baking soda, and salt.
3. In a medium bowl, whisk together melted butter and honey until smooth. Add the cinnamon, coconut milk, eggs, and apple cider vinegar, whisking together until well combined.
4. Using a spoon, stir the dry mixture into the wet mixture until thoroughly combined.
5. Scoop a large spoonful of batter into your hands and gently roll into a ball about the size of an apricot; repeat until you've made 8. Place the dough balls on a parchment-lined baking sheet two inches apart and gently flatten using the palm of your hand. (If dough is too sticky, refrigerate for about 15 minutes before rolling into balls and flattening.)
6. Bake about 15 minutes, until golden brown on top and a toothpick inserted into center comes out clean. Serve warm with a drizzle of raw honey or homemade compote.

For homemade compote: bring 1 cup blueberries, 1 Tbsp. chia seeds, and 1 Tbsp. maple syrup or honey to rolling boil. Mash with a fork and pour over biscuits.

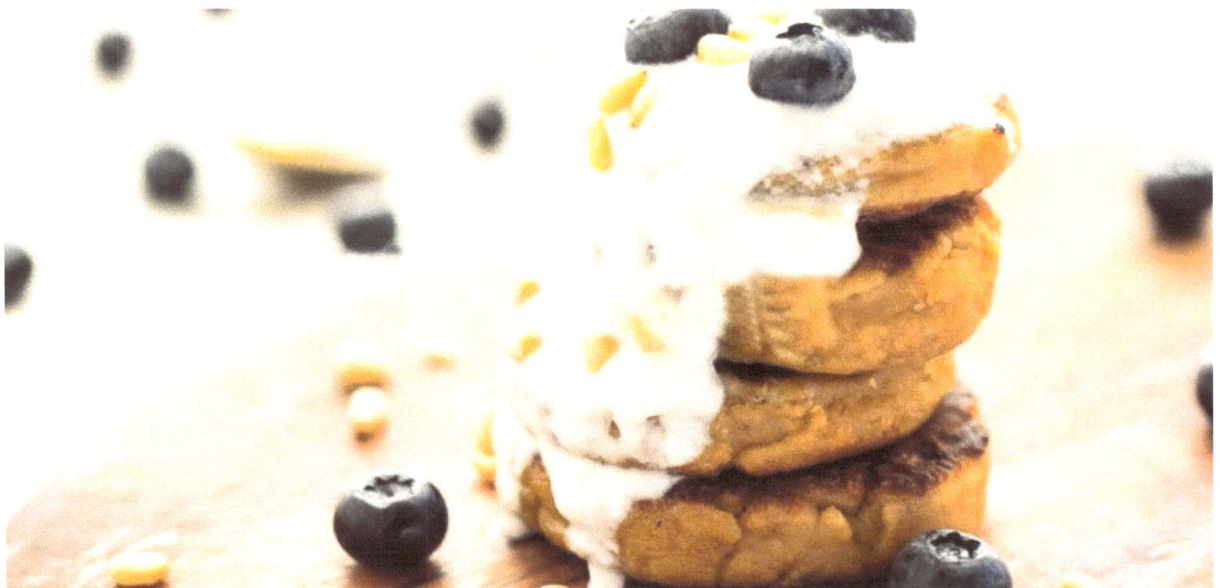

SUTTERBITES
20 servings; Prep time: 20 minutes

- ½ cup natural nut butter (options: almond, cashew, walnut at room temp.)
- 3 Tbsp. maple syrup, molasses, or honey
- 1/8 tsp. sea salt
- 2/3 cup protein powder (options: chocolate, vanilla, as long as Fattening 5 Free)
- Toppings:
- You can use any combination of these toppings!
- Unsweetened baking cocoa (cacao)
- Chia seeds, sunflower seeds
- Chocolate chunks
- Unsweetened shredded coconut
- Finely chopped pecans, walnuts, macadamias, pistachios

1) Mix all ingredients except the protein powder and blend well. Add in the protein powder.

2) Mixture should be firm, like cookie dough. Protein powders vary in consistency so if the mixture is too dry add some almond or coconut milk or some water. If it's too wet add some more protein powder, ground flaxseeds, or unsweetened baking cocoa. You have to add small amounts to get the consistency just right.

3) Scoop about 1 ½ Tbsp. and shape into a 1-inch ball.

4) Roll the ball in the toppings

5) Store in the refrigerator in airtight container

Chapter 9:

28 Day Healing Movement Map

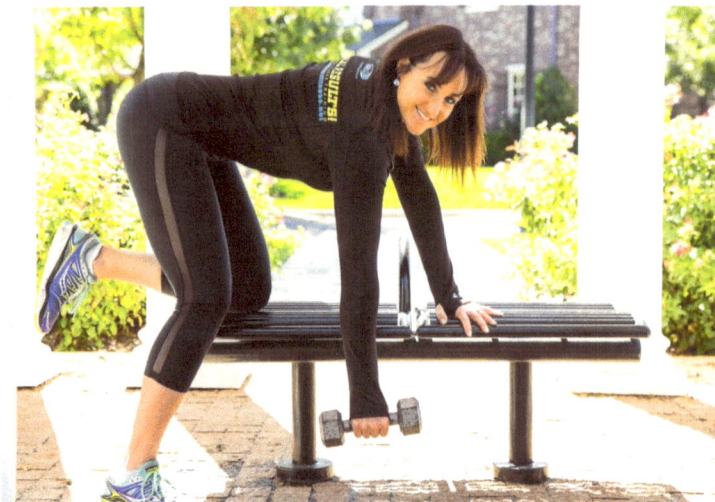

Sunday	Strength Training 20 minutes
Monday	H.I.I.T. 10 minutes
Tuesday	Gossip Walk 20 minutes
Wednesday	Strength Training 20 minutes
Thursday	Bubble Bath 30 minutes
Friday	H.I.I.T. 10 minutes
Saturday	Interval Walk

NOTES:

You must take a 3-5 minute walk break every 2 hours. Non-negotiable! You can walk circles around your desk, or walk back and forth to the restroom--just get it in.

Remember the easy weight loss benefits from Passegiata. Try to stroll for 10-20 minutes after dinner each night with the family or pets!

We do not take the weekends off with this movement map. Skipping movement on the weekends opens the door to poor food choices and the tendency to slack off and "do it later" mentality. We will stay active on the weekends!

Doctor's clearance--As with any exercise program, doctor's clearance is always recommended.

THINGS TO PURCHASE:

Stopwatch, kitchen timer or clock with a second hand Small dumbbells 3, 4, or 5 lbs

Sunday

Strength Training 20 minutes

Warm up 2 minutes with a walk or modified jumping jacks

Week 1 Goal: 1 round in 20 minutes or less

Week 2 Goal :2 rounds in 20-25 minutes

Week 3 Goal: 3 rounds in 20-25 minutes

Week 4 Goal: 4 rounds in 20-25 minutes

Keep repeating the circuit for 20 minutes, even if you don't get all the way through the entire circuit.

10 repetitions for each exercise

Triceps chair dips

Wall sits with bicep curl

Good mornings

Teapot Tips

Side Leg lifts (10 reps each side)

Lawnmowers (10 reps each arm)

Seated knee twists (or standing)

Super girls

Seated Ab Bicycles

Monday

HIIT 10 minutes

Use the first 3 exercises to increase the heart rate

Week 1 Goal: 1-2 rounds in 7 minutes

Week 2 Goal: 2-3 rounds in 7 minutes

Week 3 Goal: 3-4 rounds in 7-9 minutes

Week 4 Goal: 4-5 rounds in 7-9 minutes

After the first 3 exercises, Go HARD! Set the timer for 7 minutes. Do as many rounds as possible in 7 minutes.

1 minute per exercise

March in place

Modified Jumping Jacks

Floor to Ceilings

Set timer for 7 minutes. 15 reps per exercise.

Chair Mountain climbers

Frankenstein

Military Marchers

Rest (60 seconds, 30 seconds, 15 seconds) try to decrease rest time each week.

During rest time--don't sit. Walk in circles, step in place, keep moving.

Tuesday

Gossip Walk 15-20 minutes

Unless it is completely unbearable, do this walk outside. Bundle up if it's cold!

Week 1 Goal: 1 mile, chart time/distance

Week 2 Goal : > week 1 chart time/distance

Week 3 Goal : > week 2 chart time/distance

Week 4 Goal : > week 3 chart time/distance

Walk at a pace that you can talk but not sing. You should be breathing heavier while talking.

Wednesday

Strength Training 20 minutes

Warm up 2 minutes with a walk or modified jumping jacks

Week 1 Goal: 1 round in 20 minutes or less

Week 2 Goal :2 rounds in 20-25 minutes

Week 3 Goal: 3 rounds in 20-25 minutes

Week 4 Goal: 4 rounds in 20-25 minutes

Keep repeating the circuit for 20 minutes, even if you don't get all the way through the entire circuit.

10 repetitions for each exercise

Wall push-ups (can use sofa back)

Stand ups

Hamstring curls (10 reps each leg)

Windmills

Sumo Squats

Batmans

Russian Twists

Right X

Left X

Thursday

Bubble Bath 30 minutes

This is your Rest and Relaxation day. Spend 30 minutes on something that makes you feel good.

Massage

Nap

Pedicure/Manicure

Yoga

Friday

HIIT 10 minutes

Use the first 3 exercises to increase the heart rate

Week 1 Goal: 1-2 rounds in 7 minutes

Week 2 Goal: 2-3 rounds in 7 minutes

Week 3 Goal: 3-4 rounds in 7-9 minutes

Week 4 Goal: 4-5 rounds in 7-9 minutes

After the first 3 exercises, Go HARD! Set the timer for 7 minutes. Do as many rounds as possible in 7 minutes.

1 minute per exercise

March in place

Modified Jumping Jacks

Floor to Ceilings

Set timer for 7 minutes. 15 reps per exercise.

Big X

Tin Man

Upsy Daisy (chair step outs)

Rest (:60 seconds, :30 seconds, :15 seconds try to decrease rest time each week.

During rest time-don't sit. Walk in circles, step in place, keep moving.

SUNDAY

Strength Training **20 minutes**

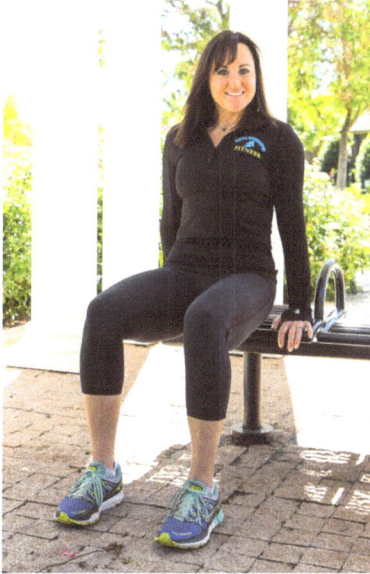

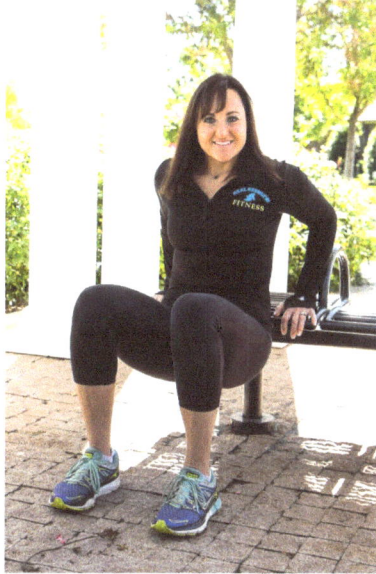

Triceps Dips

Grip chair seat with hands flat and fingers curled underneath the seat. Keep both legs at a 90-degree angle as you lower your body by bending your elbows. Keep your back as close to the chair as possible. Depth is not important, just push through your hands. Even holding this position without moving your body will work!

Wall sits with bicep curls

Stand with your back flush against the wall. Walk your feet out about 18 inches from the wall. The further your feet are away from the wall and the more weight you can put in your heels, the easier on your knees. The closer you can bring your legs to a 90-degree angle the better--but stop before any pain in your knee! Keeping your entire spine pressed into the wall, curl the dumbbells from your hips to your chest. You can do this movement without the dumbbells--just focus on squeezing the bicep.

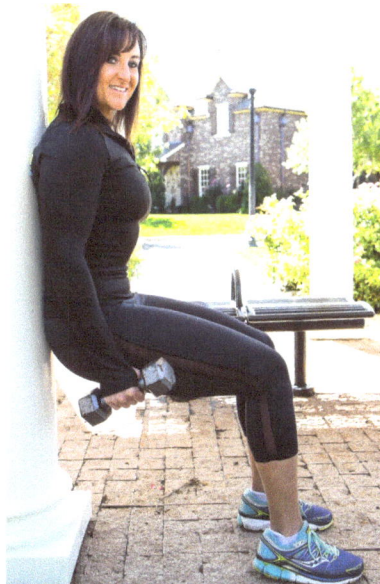

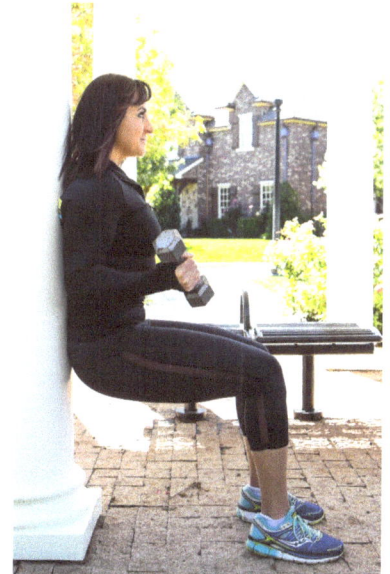

Good Mornings

This exercise should engage lower back, glutes (booty), and hamstrings (upper muscle on back of the legs). Screw the heels into the ground with toes pressing out against your shoes, cross your arms, straighten your legs, and lower yourself to hip high with a flat back, squeezing your booty and hamstrings the entire time. Reverse the motion, still squeezing the target muscles.

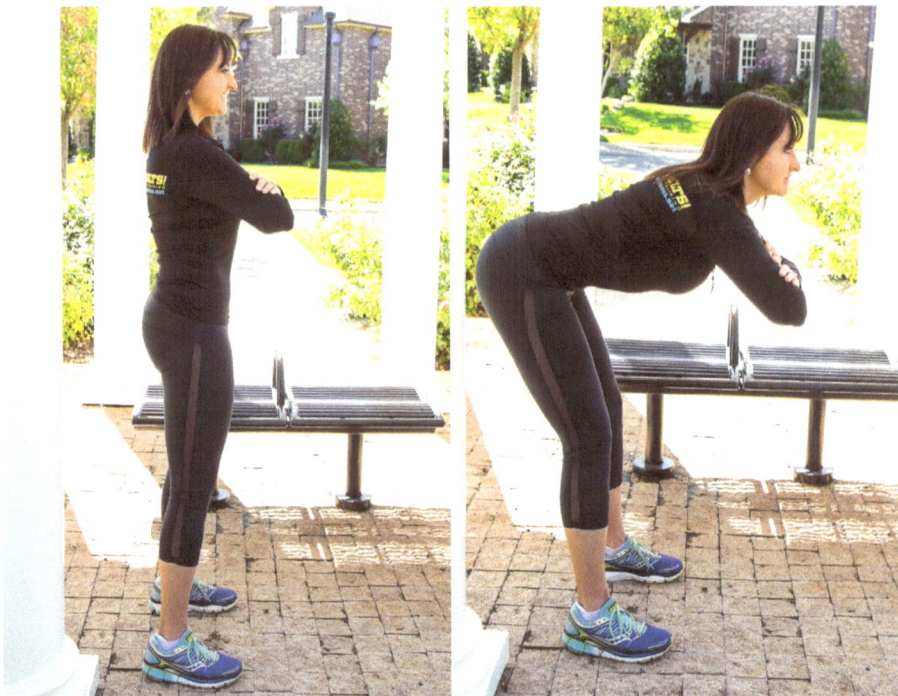

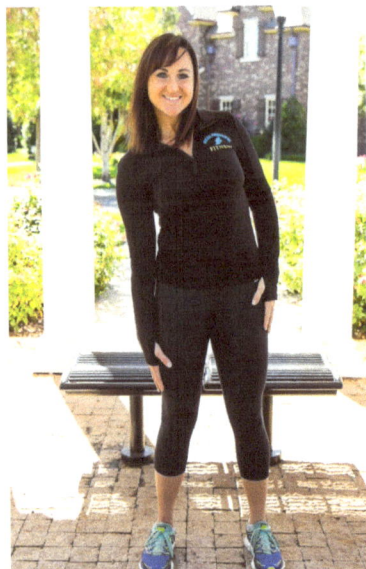

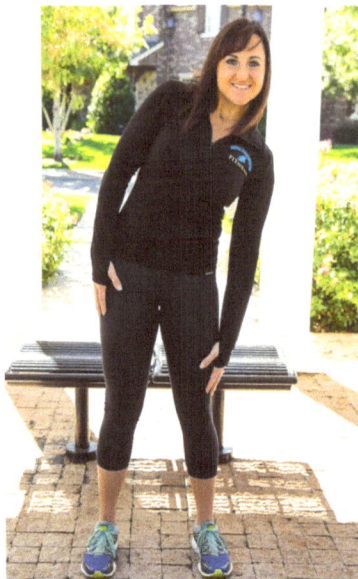

Teapot Tips

Stand with feet shoulder-width apart and both hands at your sides. Engage your abdominal wall and slide your right hand down your thigh as low as you can. Repeat on the opposite side. Think about bringing the rib cage to the hipbone.

Side Leg lifts (10 reps each side)

Use the left hand to balance on a wall if needed. Right hand on the right hip. Lift the right leg out from your side slowly as high as you can. Slowly return to the starting position. After 10 on the right leg, start with the left leg.

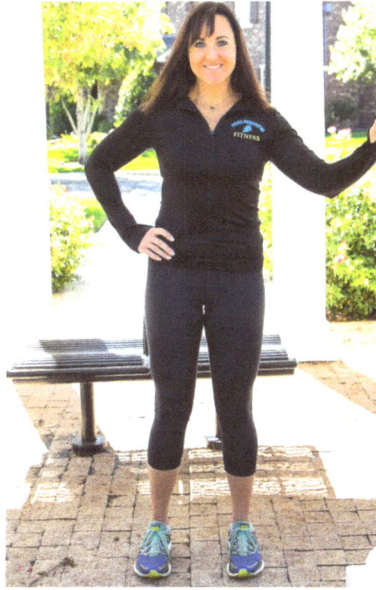

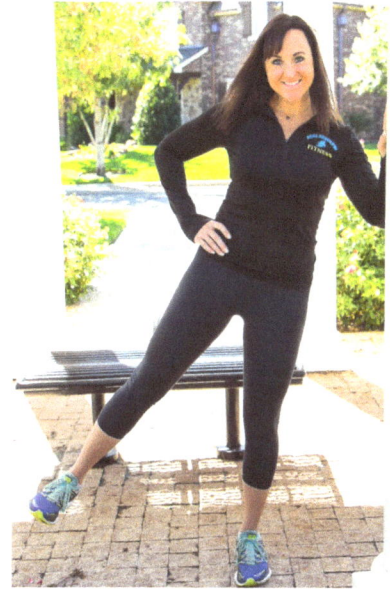

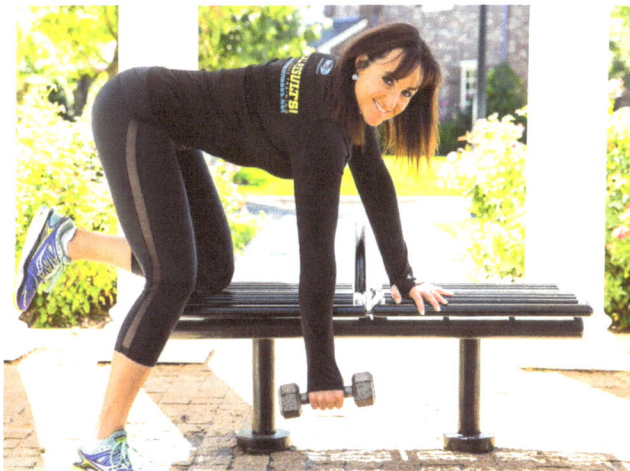

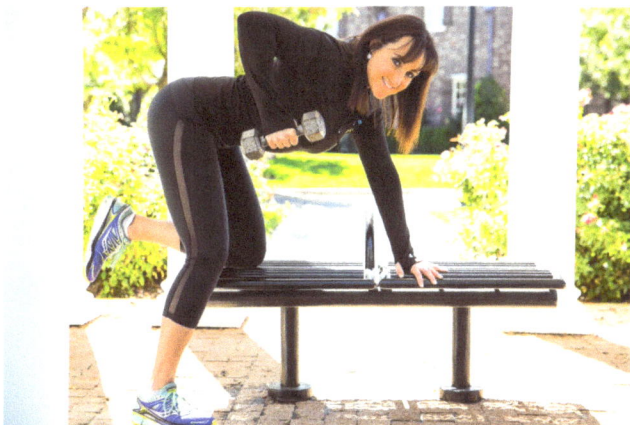

Lawnmowers (10 reps each arm)

Put the left hand and left knee on a couch or bench. Start with the right dumbbell on the floor. Grasp the dumbbell and pull it to the right armpit. Lower the dumbbell to the floor and repeat. After 10 reps, turn around on the couch and place the right hand and right knee on the couch while repeating the exercise on the left side.

Seated knee twists (or standing)

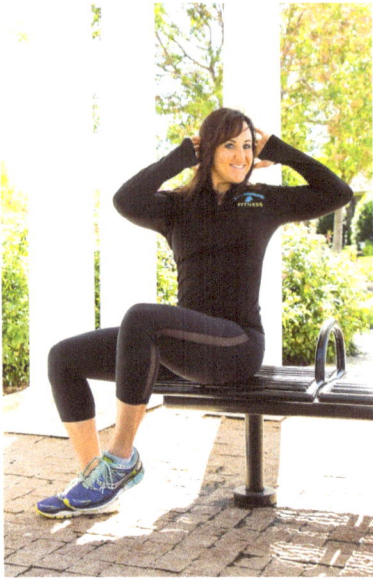

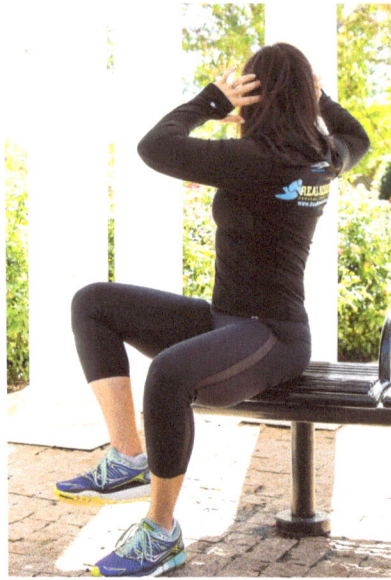

Sit in a chair with feet flat on the floor and spine straight. Engage the abdominal wall. Keeping the elbows elevated, twist the torso moving the right elbow in the direction of the left knee. Lift the left knee as the right elbow moves toward it. Do not lower the elbow to the knee. The goal is to create a twisting motion, not a crunching motion. Alternate sides. Right and left equals 1 rep.

Super girls

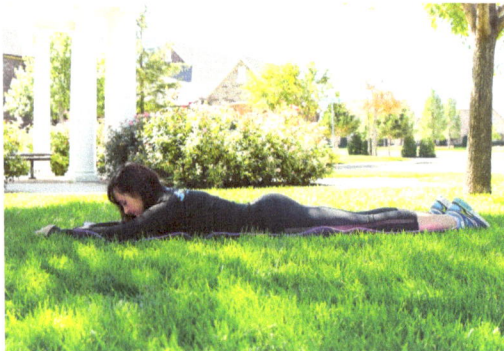

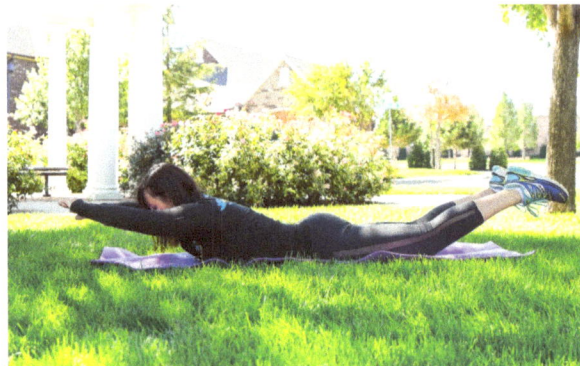

Lay on your tummy. Stretch your arms out in front. Keep your neck relaxed and head down. Raise your arms and your legs squeezing your booty. Up and down is 1 rep.

Seated Ab Crunch

Sit on the edge of a chair. Lean slightly back to engage the core muscles and hold the chair behind or on the side. Extend the legs out straight in front of you. Flex the right toe and pull the right knee into the chest. Return to start and repeat on the left side. Right and left equals 1 rep.

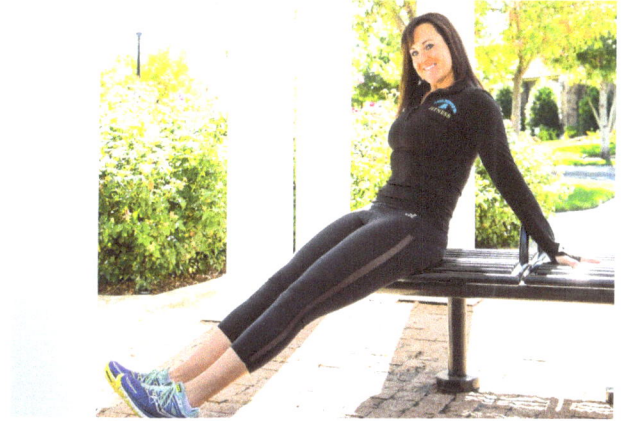

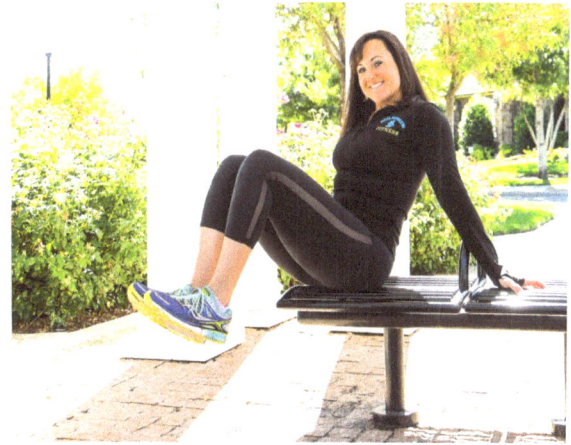

MONDAY

HIIT **10 minutes**

March in Place

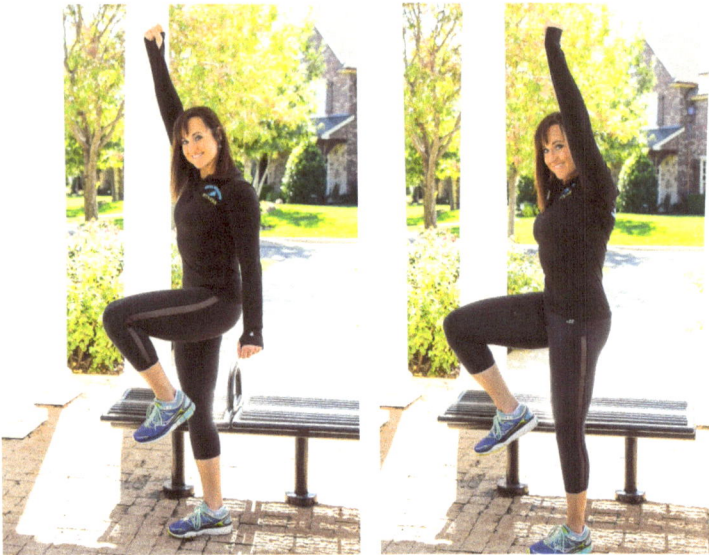

Standing upright, punch the right arm into the air above your head as you lift the left leg to a 90-degree angle. Return to start and repeat on the opposite side. Continue this motion for one minute.

Modified Jumping Jacks

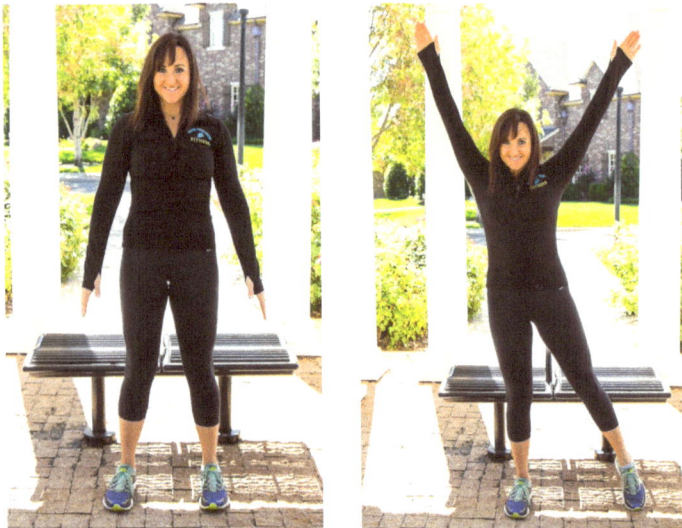

Step the right leg out to the right side as you circle both arms above your head. Return to start and repeat on the opposite side. Continue this motion for one minute.

Floor to ceilings

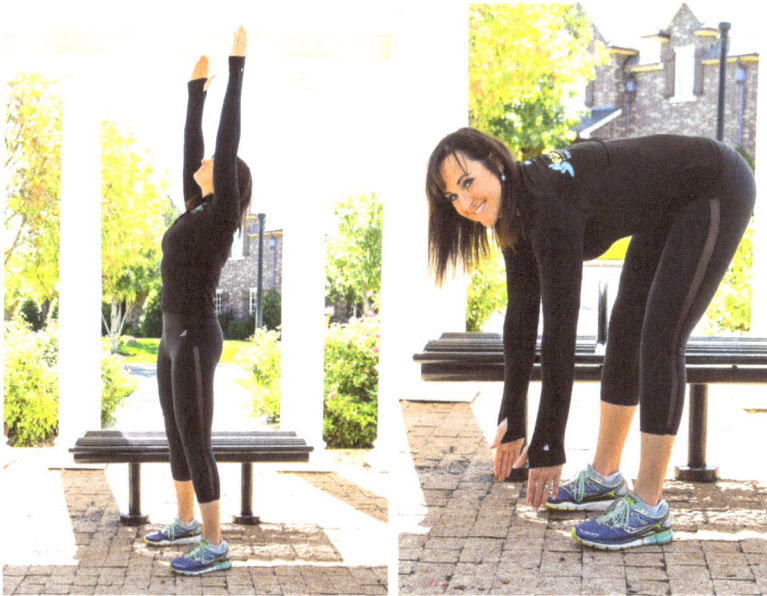

Stand with feet shoulder-width apart. Reach hands down towards the floor with straight legs and relaxed knees. Hang for one second then swing arms up and stretch up towards the ceiling. Continue this motion for one minute.

Chair Mountain climbers

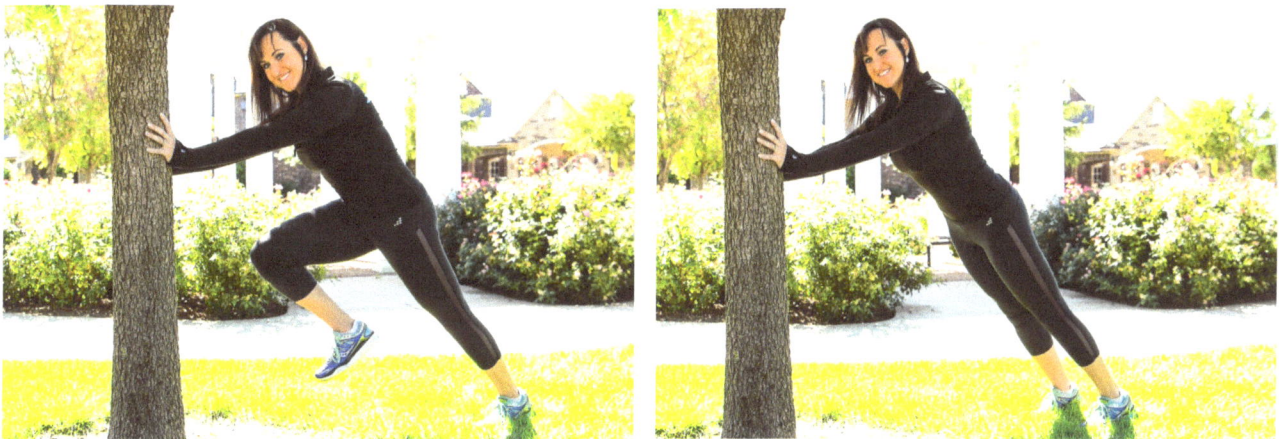

Put both hands on a chair that is pushed up against a wall. Keeping a flat back and tight abdominal wall pull the right knee into the chest. Return to start and repeat with the left knee. Right and left side is 1 rep.

Frankenstein

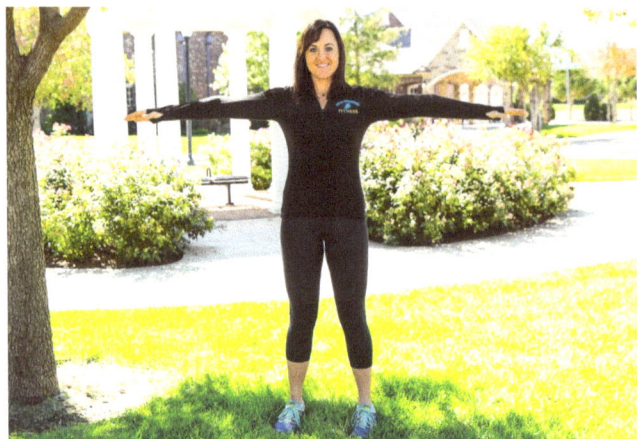

Stand upright outstretch the arms to the side shoulder height. Bring the arms together in front of your body as you raise the straightened right leg in front of you. Return to start and repeat with the left leg. Right and left side is 1 rep.

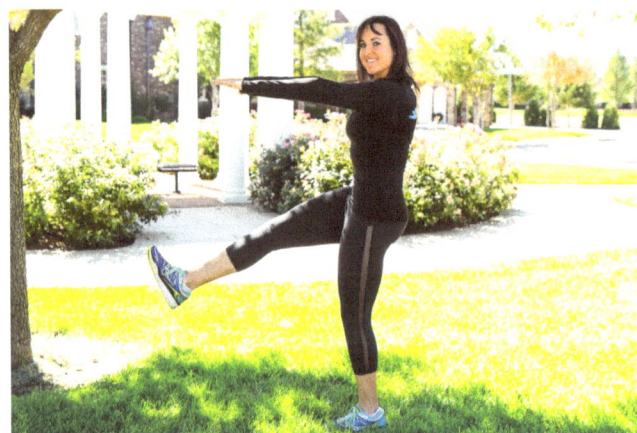

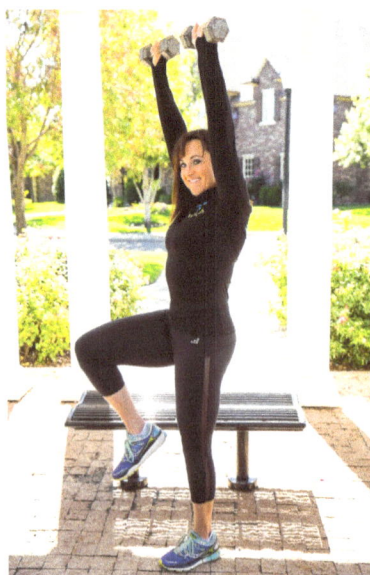

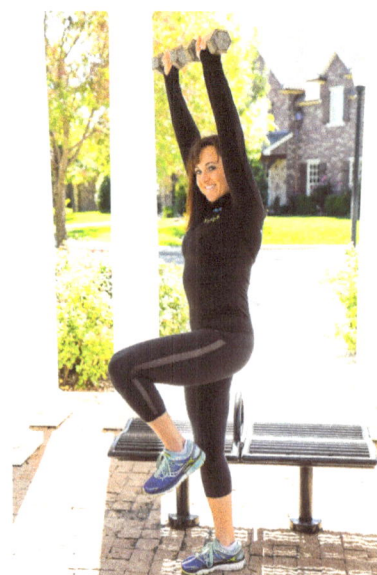

Military Marchers

Stand upright with arms at a 90-degree angle shoulder height. Press both arms above your head as you pull the right knee up to a 90-degree angle. Return to start and repeat with the left leg. Right and left side is 1 rep.

WEDNESDAY

Strength Training **20 minutes**

Wall push-ups (can use sofa back)

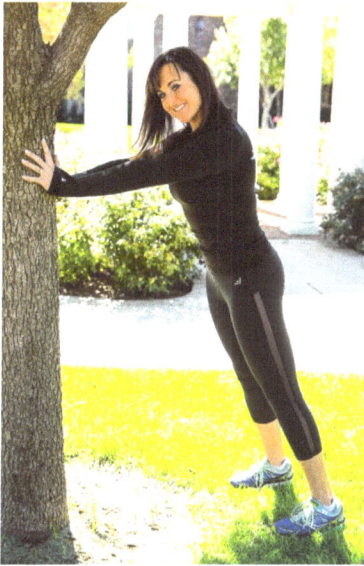

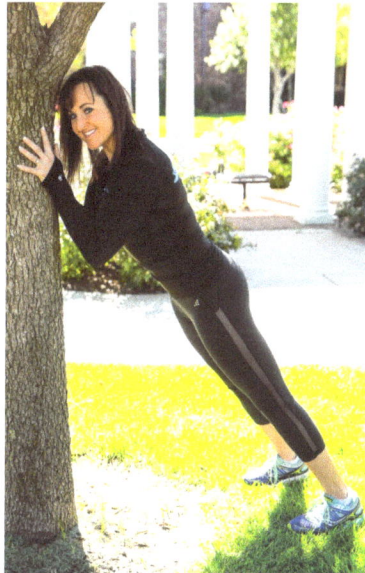

Stand about two feet away from a wall, back of a sofa, or countertop. Place hands on wall about shoulder height. Keep abdominal wall tight as you lower the chest toward the wall or sofa. Take the hips toward the wall--do not push the booty back. Push back to starting position. Each push back is 1 rep.

Stand ups

Use a supportive non-skid chair with arm rails if possible. Start sitting in the chair with feet flat. Put hands in prayer position at chest or on the arm rails. Push weight into the heels as you come to a standing position. Torso should stay straight--do not bend forward to stand up. Use the arm rails for added support if needed. After standing, push weight into heels and push booty backwards to lower yourself back into the chair. Each up and down is 1 rep.

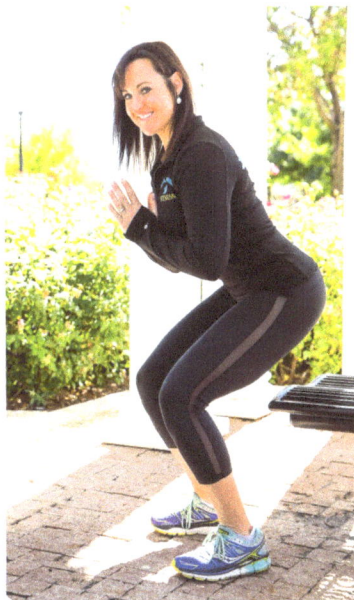

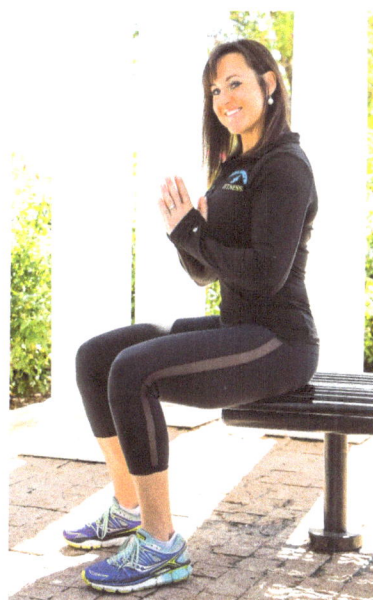

Hamstring curls
(10 reps each leg)

Stand against a wall to use for balance if necessary. Extend the left leg behind and point the toe. Squeeze the booty and hamstring (back of the leg) as you curl the heel towards the booty. Reverse the motion still squeezing the target muscles. After 10 on the left leg, start with the right leg.

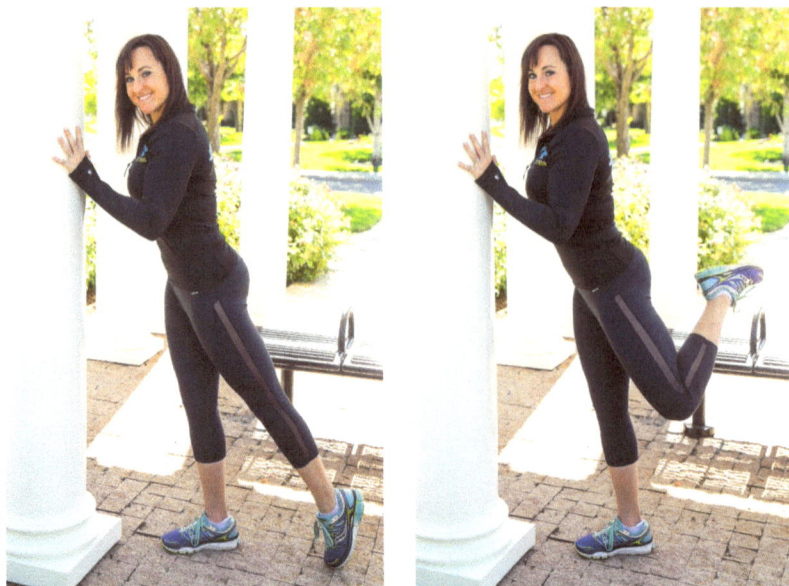

Windmills

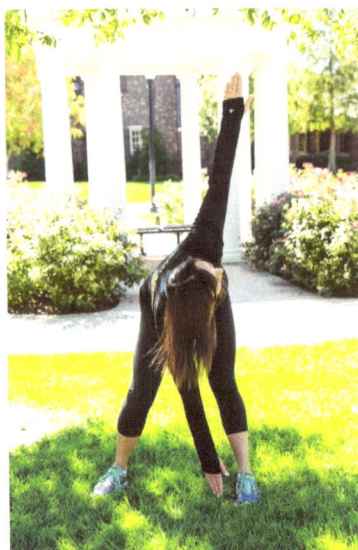

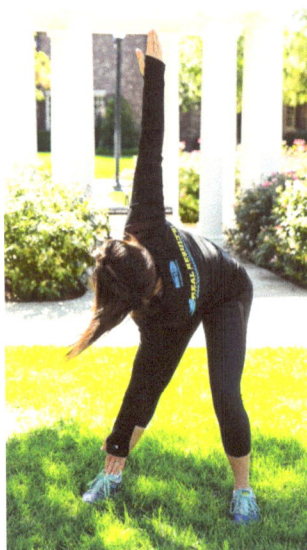

Stand with feet wider than hip width, and both arms extended out to sides, shoulder height with pointed fingers. Take the right hand down towards the left toe with the left hand extended up to the ceiling. Pause then return to start. Repeat motion on opposite side. Right and left side is 1 rep.

Sumo Squats

Take feet much wider than hip width and turn the toes out as far as possible. Press the weight into the heels and squeeze the booty. Allow the knees to track outward as you lower your body as close to a 90 degree as possible. *If you track the knees out there should be no knee pain. Hold for one second then return to start. Up and down is 1 rep.

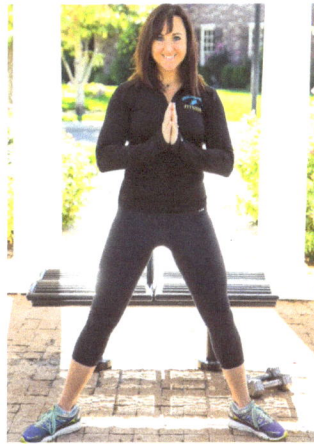

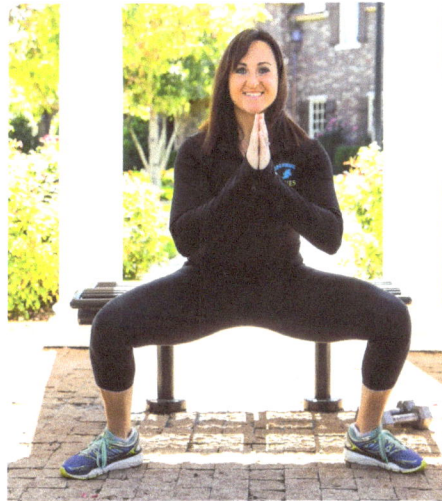

Batmans

Soften the knees and flatten the back to hip high. Grasp a dumbbell in each hand and hanging about knee high. Slightly bend the elbows as you fly both arms up to shoulder height. Stay in squat position the entire time. Without dumbbells think about squeezing the upper back and arms. Up and down is 1 rep.

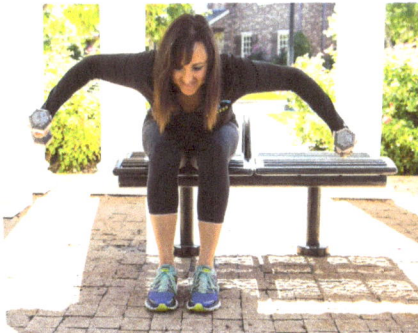

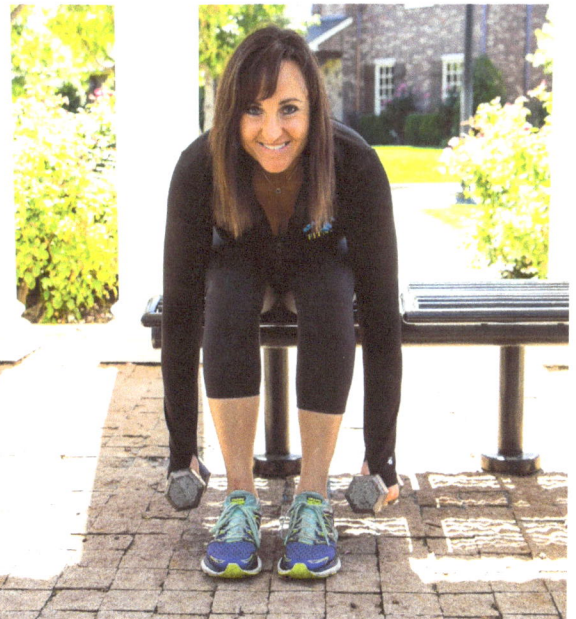

Scarecrows

Standing with feet shoulder width apart arms up at 90-degree angles hold dumbbells if possible. Tip the body to the left side focusing on bringing the ribcage towards the hipbone. Return to start and repeat on the other side. Focus on crunching the core, not dropping the shoulders. Right side and left side is 1 rep.

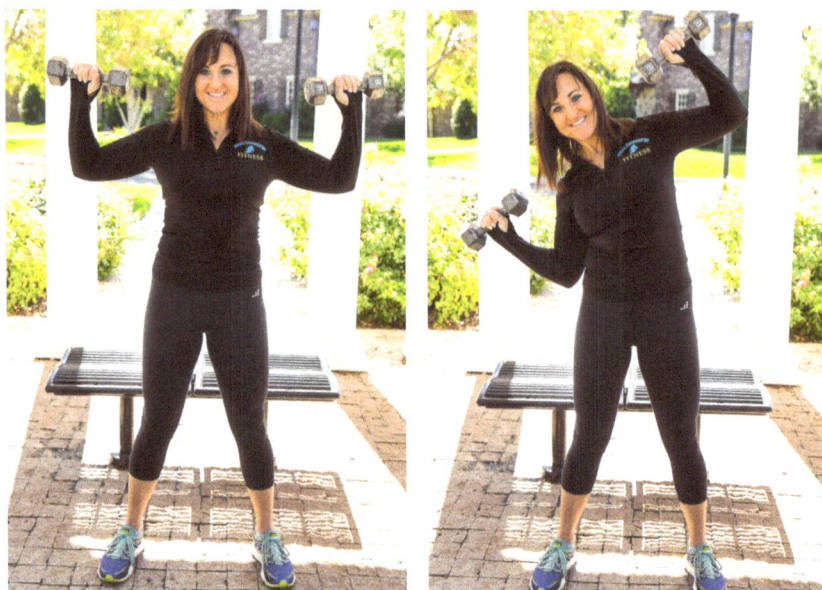

Core Xs

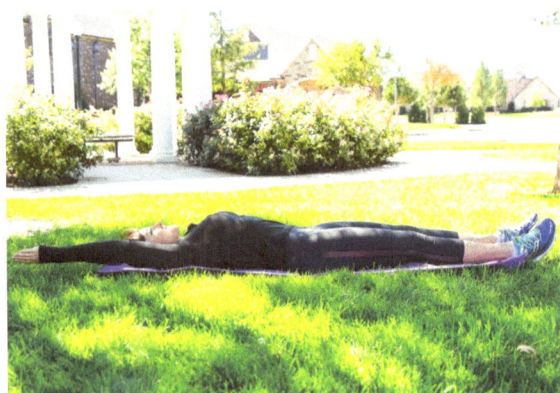

Lay on your back with right arm stretched behind you, left arm at side, and both legs straight. Reach the right arm and left leg towards each other and meet in the middle. Return to start and repeat with opposite side. Right and left is 1 rep.

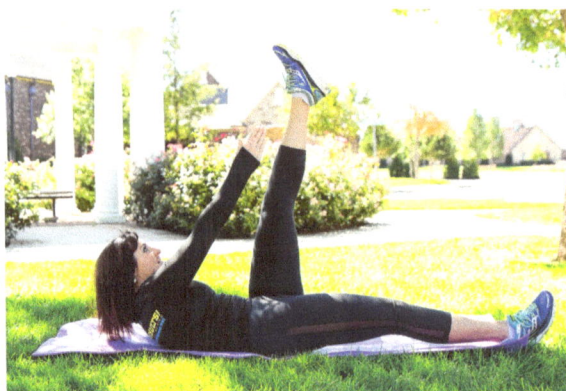

Heel taps

Standing tall with feet hip width apart raise the right foot and tap the right heel with the left hand. Focus on tightening the abdominal wall and standing tall. Return to start and repeat on opposite side. Right and left is 1 rep.

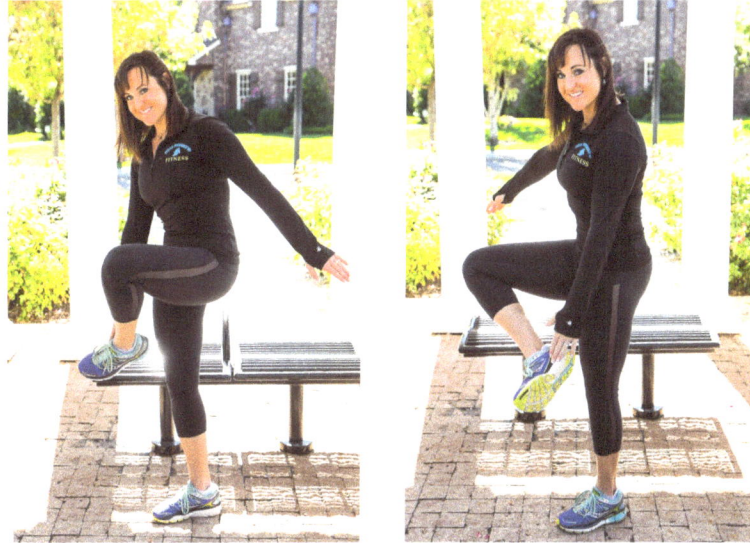

HIIT **10 minutes**

Big X

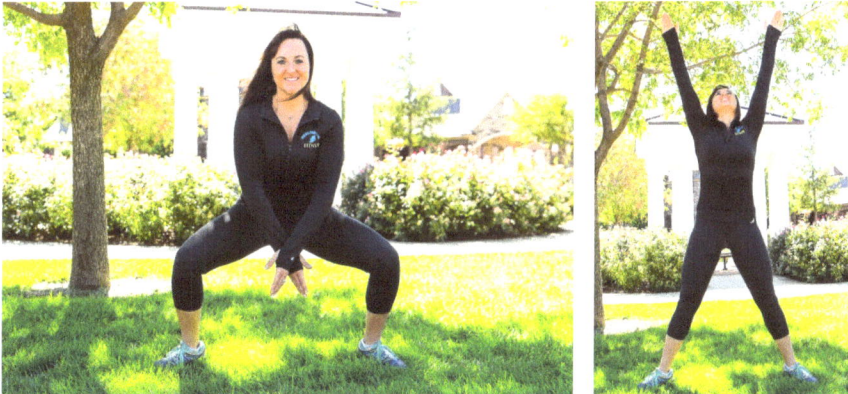

Stand in sumo squat position, with feet outside hip width and toes turned out. Track the knees out as you sweep both arms down towards the ground. Cross the arms in the middle and then sweep them up and over head, crossing in the middle overhead. Continue this motion for one minute.

Tin Man

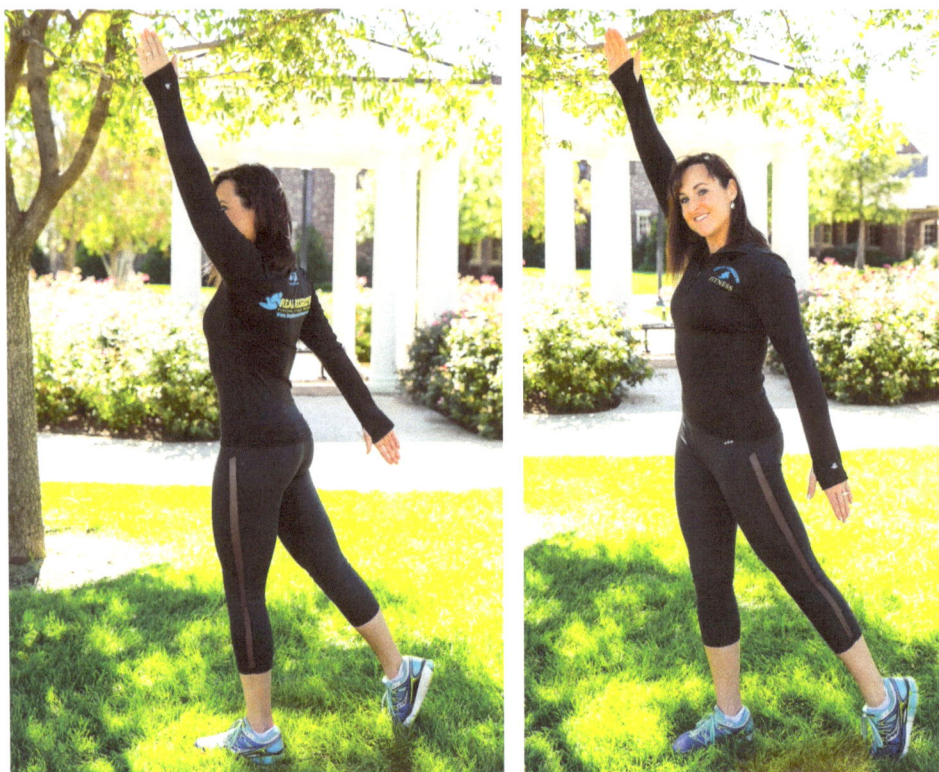

Start with the left leg behind on the toe, and the right arm stretched overhead. Sweep the right arm down to your side as you raise the left arm. Step the left leg forward as you step the right leg backwards. Focus on engaged abdominal wall and tall straight spine. Continue this motion for one minute.

Upsy Daisy (chair step outs)

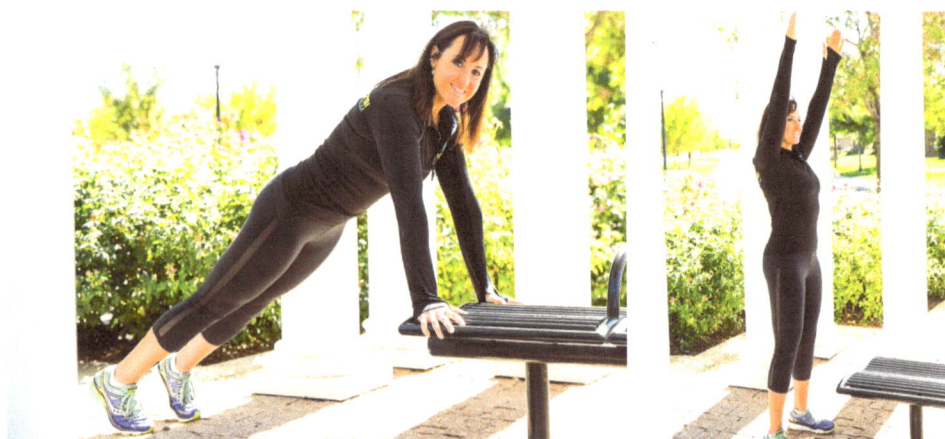

Use a supportive non-skid chair. Standing six inches from the chair, bend down and place both hands on the chair. Step the right foot back then the left foot back. Hold this plank position for one second. Step the right foot in and the left foot in and stand up. Continue this motion for one minute.

Chapter 10:

Weekly **Meal Planner**

Date: Week 1

Weekday	Breakfast	Snack 1	Lunch	Snack 2	Dinner
S	Sunrise Shake	Jessica's Jazzy Trail mix	Turkey Berry Colorful Salad	Chocolate Chip Cookie Dough	2 ingredient Italian chicken, 2 cups mixed spring greens, and 1 cup sautéed zucchini
M	Good Morning Burrito	Bullet-proof Coffee	Chicken in Berry Colorful Salad	Good Morning Burrito	Spicy Salmon, 2 cups baby romaine
T	Choco Covered Cherry Smoothie	Jessica's Jazzy Trail mix	Salmon Berry Colorful Salad	Chocolate Chip Cookie Dough	Beef Fajitas
W	Mexican Egg Omelet	Bullet-proof Coffee	Beef Berry Colorful Salad	Mexican Egg Omelet	Passing Lane: 2 ingredient Italian chicken, 2 cups mixed spring greens, and 1 cup sautéed zucchini
T	Sunrise Shake	Jessica's Jazzy Trail mix	Turkey Berry Colorful Salad	Chocolate Chip Cookie Dough	Passing Lane: Spicy Salmon, 2 cups baby romaine
F	Good Morning Burrito	Bullet-proof Coffee	Deli Chicken Berry Colorful Salad	Good Morning Burrito	Passing Lane: Beef Fajitas
S	Choco Covered Cherry Smoothie	Jessica's Jazzy Trail mix	Scenic Route Lunch!	Chocolate Chip Cookie Dough	Clean Eating Restaurant of Choice

Weekly **Meal Planner**

Date: Week 2

Weekday	Breakfast	Snack 1	Lunch	Snack 2	Dinner
S	Jessica McMuffin	Sutter-Bites	Sunday Roast with paleo biscuits	Jessica Mc-Muffin	2 ingredient Salmon Boats
M	Pump-kin Spice Latte	Paleo Biscuits w blueberry compote	Salmon Nutty but Nice Salad	Apple & 2 tbsp. Al-mond butter	Roasted Ranch Chick-en, roasted carrots, on-ions, zucchini, okra
T	Sunrise Shake	Sutter-Bites	Chicken Nutty but Nice Salad	Carrots & 2 tbsp. Hum-mus	Meat Only Meatloaf
W	Mexican Egg Om-elet	Paleo Biscuits w blueberry compote	Roast Nutty but Nice Salad	Mexican Egg Omelet	Passing Lane:- 2 ingredient Salmon Boats
T	Pump-kin Spice Latte	Sutter-Bites	Turkey Nutty but Nice Salad	Apple & 2 tbsp. Al-mond butter	Passing Lane: Roasted Ranch Chick-en, roasted carrots, on-ions, zucchini, okra
F	Jessica McMuffin	Paleo Biscuits w blueberry compote	Deli Chicken Nutty but Nice Salad	Jessica Mc-Muffin	Passing Lane: Meat Only Meatloaf
S	Sunrise Shake	Sutter-Bites	Scenic Route Lunch!	Carrots & 2 tbsp. Hum-mus	Clean Eating Restaurant of Choice

Weekly **Meal Planner**

Date: Week 3

Weekday	Breakfast	Snack 1	Lunch	Snack 2	Dinner
S	Sunrise Shake	Jessica's Jazzy Trail mix	Sunday Ham w/ Side Salad	Chocolate Chip Cookie Dough	Melt in Your Mouth Chicken
M	Good Morning Burrito	Bullet-proof Coffee	Jessica's Ham-wich	Good Morning Burrito	Tuna Patty with Personality
T	Choco Covered Cherry Smoothie	Jessica's Jazzy Trail mix	MYM Chicken in lettuce wraps	Carrots & 2 tbsp. Hummus	Mexican Chicken
W	Mexican Egg Omelet	Bullet-proof Coffee	Tuna in lettuce wraps	Mexican Egg Omelet	Passing Lane: Melt in Your Mouth Chicken
T	Sunrise Shake	Jessica's Jazzy Trail mix	Jessica's Ham-wich	Chocolate Chip Cookie Dough	Passing Lane: Mexican Chicken
F	Good Morning Burrito	Bullet-proof Coffee	Mexican chicken in lettuce wraps	Good Morning Burrito	Passing Lane: Tuna Patty w/ Personality
S	Choco Covered Cherry Smoothie	Jessica's Jazzy Trail mix	Scenic Route Lunch!	Apple & 2 tbsp. Almond Butter	Clean Eating Restaurant of Choice

Weekly **Meal Planner**

Date: Week 4

Weekday	Breakfast	Snack 1	Lunch	Snack 2	Dinner
S	Jessica McMuffin	Sutter-Bites	Sunday Roast with paleo biscuits	Jessica Mc-Muffin	Portabella Cheeseburger
M	Pump-kin Spice Latte	Paleo Biscuits w blueberry compote	Shredded Roast in Bell Peppers	Carrots & 2 tbsp. Hum-mus	BBQ chicken Lettuce wraps
T	Sunrise Shake	Sutter-Bites	BBQ Chicken wraps	Bliss Bar	Orange Chicken
W	Mexican Egg Om-elet	Paleo Biscuits w blueberry compote	Orange chick-en wraps	Mexican Egg Omelet	Passing Lane: Portabella Cheeseburger
T	Pump-kin Spice Latte	Sutter-Bites	Shredded Roast in Bell Peppers	Bliss Bar	Passing Lane: BBQ chicken wraps
F	Jessica McMuffin	Paleo Biscuits w blueberry compote	Portabella Cheeseburger	Jessica Mc-Muffin	Passing Lane: Orange Chick-en
S	Sunrise Shake	Sutter-Bites	Scenic Route Lunch!	Bliss Bar	Clean Eating Restaurant of Choice

All dinners include a mixed salad unless otherwise specified.

- Cook 3 meals: 2-Ingredient Italian chicken, Spicy Salmon, Beef Fajitas

- Make Crockpot Roast for Sunday lunch

- Make 2 snacks that will last the whole month! Store them in the freezer for future use: Chocolate chip cookie dough and Jessica's Jazzy Trail Mix

- Most of the items on the staple list is for the entire 28 days.

Produce	Amount
Fresh salsa or Pico de Gallo	24 oz
Hemp Hearts shelled	1 bag
Spring Mix or Half and Half	3 boxes
Zucchini	1
Cabbage leaf or romaine leaf	3 leaves each
Chia Seeds	4 oz
Avocado or mini wholly guacamole pkgs	3 or 4 pkgs
Minced garlic or dried garlic	1 jar
Yellow onion	1
Bell peppers any color	3
Mushrooms	1 sm pkg
Asparagus	5 spears
Jalapeno, small (optional)	1
Cilantro fresh (optional)	1 bag

Pantry Staples	Amount
Clean vanilla protein powder	32 oz
Clean chocolate protein powder	32 oz
Clean fajita seasoning mix	1 pkg
Coconut/Almond milk unsweet	½ gallon
Nuts-raw (cashews, almonds, walnuts and/or pecans	10 cups
Unsweet coconut flakes	5 cups
65% or higher dark chocolate	3 cups
Balsamic Vinegar	1 bottle
Lime juice (no additives)	1 bottle
Italian herb spaghetti sauce	25 oz
Coconut spray for skillets	1 bottle
Unrefined virgin expeller pressed coconut oil	1 jar
Coffee, chai tea, or alternative	3+ cups
Extra Virgin Olive oil	16oz
Spices/seasonings in small jars or bags:	
Liquid stevia, Vanilla extract, Celtic sea salt, black pepper, cinnamon, onion salt, cayenne	
Natural Almond Butter (or PB)	24 oz jar
Oat Flour	2 cups
Maple Syrup (pure)	16 oz
Honey (raw)	16 oz
Baking cocoa	½ cup
Paleo Mayo	16 oz
Apple Cider Vinegar	1 sm bottle

Proteins	Amount
Clean Deli turkey	8 oz
Clean Deli chicken	8 oz
Chicken breasts	4, 6 oz
Farm or omega 3 eggs	dozen
Organic butter	2 sticks
Salmon frozen or fresh	4, 6 oz
Kefir or Yogurt plain unsweet	1 cup
Flank Steak	1.5 lbs
Block Cheese of choice	2 cups
Chuck Roast	2-3lbs

Fruit	Amount
Blueberries	7 cups frozen or fresh
Cherries	2 cups frozen or fresh

Week 2: Meal Prep and Planning

- Cook 3 meals: 2-Ingredient Salmon Boats, Roasted Ranch Chicken, Meat Only Meatloaf

- Make Oven Ham for Sunday lunch

- Make 2 snacks that will last the whole month! Store them in the freezer for future use: Paleo Biscuits and SutterBites

Produce	Amount
Fresh salsa or Pico de Gallo	8 oz
Baby Spinach	6 cups
Spring Mix or Half and Half	3 boxes
Zucchini	1
Carrots, baby	1 pkg
Okra	12 pods
Green onions	3
Avocado or mini wholly guacamole pkgs	1 or 2 pkgs
Green beans or Brussel sprouts	16 oz
Yellow onion	2
Bell peppers any color	3
Hummus	6 oz
Jalapeno, small (optional)	1
Cilantro fresh (optional)	1 bag

Proteins	Amount
Clean Deli turkey	8 oz
Clean Deli chicken	8 oz
Chicken breasts	8, 6 oz
Clean and natural bacon	2 lbs
Farm or omega 3 eggs	1 dozen
Tuna canned in water	3, 6 oz cans
(Kefir or Yogurt plain unsweet	1 cup
Block Cheese of choice	2 cups
Chuck Roast	2-3lbs
Organic butter	3 Tbsp

Pantry Staples	Amount
Sunflower Seeds, raw unsalted	1 cup
Aluminum foil or alternativ	1 box
Clean ranch seasoning mix	2 pkgs
Coconut/Almond milk unsweet	½ gallon
Chicken broth (Fattening 5 free)	1 cup
Pumpkin canned (plain)	1 can
Pumpkin pie spice (optional)	1 jar
Blanched Almond flour	5 cups
Coffee	20 oz

Fruit	Amount
Blueberries	2 cups
Apples	2

Week 3: Meal Prep and Planning

- Cook 3 meals: Tuna Patty with Personality, Melt in Your Mouth Chicken, Mexican Chicken
- Make Sunday crockpot Roast

Produce	Amount
Fresh salsa or Pico de Gallo	20 oz
Baby Spinach	6 cups
Spring Mix or Half and Half	3 boxes
Butter lettuce, cabbage, or romaine leaf	12 leaves
Carrots, baby	1 pkg
Pickles for Hamwich (no colors or additives)	1 jar
Avocado or mini wholly guacamole pkgs	2 or 3 pkgs
Yellow onion	2
Bell peppers any color	1
Mushrooms	1 small pkg
Hummus (check pantry)	6 oz
Jalapeno, small (optional)	1
Cilantro fresh (optional)	1 bag
Minced garlic (check pantry)	1 jar

Fruit	Amount
Blueberries	1 cup
Apples	1
Cherries	2 cups

Proteins	Amount
Clean Deli turkey	8 oz
Clean Deli chicken	8 oz
Chicken breasts	8, 6 oz
Clean and natural bacon	2 lbs
Farm or omega 3 eggs	1 dozen
Tuna canned in water cans (che	3, 6 oz
Kefir or Yogurt plain unsweet	1 cup
Block Cheese of choice	2 cups
Chuck Roast	2-3lbs
Organic butter	3 Tbsp

Pantry Staples	Amount
Paleo Mayo (check pantry)	2 cups
Clean ranch seasoning mix	1 pkg
Clean taco seasoning mix	1 pkg
Spices to consider:	1 pkg each cumin, ginger, cayenne
Coconut/Almond milk unsweet	½ gallon
Nut butter (check pantry)	1 jar
Coffee	20 oz
65%-100% dark chocolate	2 cups

- Cook 3 meals: Hamburger on Portabella, Crockpot BBQ Chicken Lettuce Wraps, Crockpot Orange Chicken

- Make Bliss bar snacks

Produce	Amount
Fresh salsa or Pico de Gallo	6 oz
Baby Spinach	6 cups
Spring Mix or Half and Half	3 boxes
Leafy lettuce	1 bunch
Carrots, baby	1 pkg
Portabella mushroom caps	4-6 caps
Avocado or mini wholly guacamole pkgs	2 or 3 pkgs
Yellow and red onion	1 each
Bell peppers any color	2
Tomatoes	1
Green chilis (optional)	1 jar
Hummus (check pantry)	6 oz
Jalapeno, small (optional)	1
Cilantro fresh (optional)	1 bag

Proteins	Amount
Ground beef	2.5 lbs
Chicken breasts	8, 6 oz
Farm or omega 3 eggs	4 eggs
Kefir or Yogurt plain unsweet	1 cup

Pantry Staples	Amount
Clean BBQ sauce, low sugar	16 oz
Pumpkin seeds	½ cup
Ground Flax seed	½ cup
Coconut/Almond milk unsweet	½ gallon
Nut butter (check pantry)	1 jar
Coconut Aminos	1 sm bottle
Pumpkin canned (plain)	1 cup
Orange Juice	½ cup
Sesame oil (can use olive oil instead)	

Fruit	Amount
Blueberries	2 cups

BIBLIOGRAPHY

_____

MEET YOUR SIRI

Stein, Skip."Genetics Loads the Gun, Lifestyle Pulls the Trigger."Journal of Nutritional Health Food Engineering 3, no. 2 (December 2015). Accessed July 10, 2017. doi: 10.15406/jnhfe.2015.03.00107.

Chapter 4

Pedersen, Bente K. "Muscle-to-Fat Interaction: ATwo-way Street?" Journal of Physiology 588(January 2010). Accessed September 3, 2017. doi: 10.1113/jphysiol.2009.184747.

Seebohar,Bob. Metabolic Efficiency Training: Teaching the Body to Burn More Fat, 2nd ed. N.p.: Fuel4mance, 2014.

Chapter 5

American Diabetes Association. "Glycemic Index and Diabetes." May 14, 2014. Accessed September 15, 2017. http://www.diabetes.org/food-and-fitness/food/what-can-i-eat/understanding-carbohydrates/glycemic-index-and-diabetes.html?referrer=https://www.google.com/.

Bian,Xiaoming,et al. "The Artificial Sweetener Acesulfame Potassium Affects the Gut Microbiome and Body Weight Gain in CD-1 mice." PLOS ONE 12, no. 6 (June 2017). Accessed September 14, 2017. https://doi.org/10.1371/journal.pone.0178426.

Boonnate, Piyanard, et al. "Monosodium Glutamate Dietary Consumption Decreases Pancreatic β-Cell Mass in Adult Wistar Rats." PLOS ONE 10, no. 6 (June 2015). Accessed September 15, 2017. doi: 10.1371/journal.pone.0131595.

Cong, W. N., et al. "Long-term Artificial Sweetener AcesulfamePotassium Treatment Alters Neurometabolic Functions in C57BL/6J Mice." PLOS ONE 8, no. 8 (August 2013). Accessed September 14, 2017. doi: 10.1371/journal.pone.0070257.

Deol, Poonamjot, et al. "Soybean Oil Is More Obesogenic and Diabetogenic than Coconut Oil and Fructose in Mouse: Potential Role for the Liver." PLOS ONE 10, no. 7 (July 2015). Accessed September 14, 2017. https://doi.org/10.1371/journal.pone.0132672.

He, K., et al. "Consumption of Monosodium Glutamate in Relation to Incidence of Overweight in Chinese Adults: China Health and Nutrition Survey (CHNS) 123."American Journal of Clinical Nutrition 93, no. 6

(June 2011). Accessed September 15, 2017. doi: 10.3945/ajcn.110.008870.   122

McCall, Becky. "Artificial Sweeteners Alter Gut Response to Glucose." Medscape.Last modified September 20, 2017. Accessed Sept 30, 2017. http://www.medscape.com/viewarticle/885945.

Mercola, Joseph. "MSG: Is This Silent Killer Lurking in Your Cabinets." Mercola. Last modified April 21, 2009. Accessed September 15, 2017. http://articles.mercola.com/sites/articles/archive/2009/04/21/msg-is-this-silent-killer-lurking-in-your-kitchen-cabinets.aspx.

Mercola, Joseph. "New Study of Splenda (Sucralose) Reveals Shocking Information About Potential Harmful Effects." Mercola. Last modified February 9, 2010. Accessed September 14, 2017. http://articles.mercola.com/sites/articles/archive/2009/02/10/new-study-of-splenda-reveals-shocking-information-about-potential-harmful-effects.aspx.

Mercola, Joseph. "Soybean Oil: One of the Most Harmful Ingredients in Processed Foods." Mercola.Last modified January 27, 2013. Accessed September 14, 2017. http://articles.mercola.com/sites/articles/archive/2013/01/27/soybean-oil.aspx.

Rosenthal, Joshua. Integrative Nutrition: Feed Your Hunger for Health and Happiness, 3rd ed.N.p.: Integrative Nutrition Publishing, 2014.

Zeratsky, Katherine. "What is MSG? Is it Bad for You?" The Mayo Clinic. March 13, 2015. Accessed September 15, 2017. http://www.mayoclinic.org/healthy-lifestyle/nutrition-and-healthy-eating/expert-answers/monosodium-glutamate/faq-20058196.

Chapter 6

Feldman, D., Pike, J. W., and Adams, J. S., eds.Vitamin D, 3rded.Elsevier, UK: Academic Press, 2011. Accessed September 11, 2017.https://www.vitamindcouncil.org/about-vitamin-d/what-is-vitamin-d/.

Chapter 7

American Diabetes Association. "Sleep Duration as a Risk Factor for the Development of Type 2 Diabetes."Diabetes Care29, no. 3 (March 2006).Accessed June 5, 2017. https://doi.org/10.2337/diacare.29.03.06.dc05-0879.

Andrade, A. M., G. W. Greene,and K. J.Melanson. "Eating Slowly Led to Decreases in Energy Intake within Meals in Healthy Women." Journal of the American Dietetic Association108, no. 7 (July 2008). Accessed July 6, 2017. doi: 10.1016/j.jada.2008.04.026.

Azad, M., et al."Nonnutritive Sweeteners and Cardiometabolic Health: ASystematic Review and Meta-analysis of Randomized Controlled Trials and Prospective Cohort Studies."Canadian Medical Association Journal 189, no. 28 (July 2017). Accessed July 10, 2017. doi: 10.1503/cmaj.161390CMAJ.

Bernard, M., et al. "Breaking Sitting with Light Activities vs Structured Exercise: ARandomisedCrossover

Study Demonstrating Benefits for GlycaemicControl and Insulin Sensitivity in Type 2 Diabetes." Diabetologia60, no. 3 (March 2016). Accessed July 17, 2017. https://doi.org/10.1007/s0012

Boyles, Salynn. "Drinking Water May Speed Weight Loss: Metabolic Rate Increases Slightly with Water Consumption." WebMD. Last modified January 5, 2004. Accessed July 29, 2017. www.webmd.com/diet/news/20040105/drinking-water-may-speed-weight-loss.

Brown, Dixie.. "Binge Eating and Binge Drinking: Same Origins" Binge Eating Disorder Association,April 5, 2016. Accessed Sept 3, 2017. https://bedaonline.com/binge-eating-and-binge-drinking-same-origins/.

Buettner, Dan. *The Blue Zones: Lessons for Living Longer from the People Who've Lived the Longest.* Washington, DC: National Geographic Society, 2009.

"Comparing the Somatic and Autonomic Nervous Systems." Lumen. Accessed July 29, 2017. https://courses.lumenlearning.com/boundless-ap/chapter/introduction-to-the-autonomic-nervous-system/.

"Consequences of Insufficient Sleep Consequences of Insufficient Sleep."Healthy Sleep. Harvard Medical School. Accessed June 5, 2017. http://healthysleep.med.harvard.edu/healthy/matters/consequences.

Dennis, E. A., et al. "Water Consumption Increases Weight Loss During a Hypocaloric Diet Intervention in Middle-aged and Older Adults." Obesity 18, no. 2 (February 2011). Accessed July 29, 2017. doi: 10.1038/oby.2009.235.

Fernau, Karen. "Portion Control is in the Palm of Your Hands."USA Today, April 17, 2013. Accessed June 6, 2017.
https://www.usatoday.com/story/news/nation/2013/04/17/health-food-portion-control/2091865/.

Goff, Ronnie. "Passeggiata to Prevent Diabetes." Awaken Health Fitness. Last modified January 1, 2016. Accessed June 10, 2016. http://awakenhealthfitness.com/passeggiata-prevent-diabetes/

Holla, Anand. "The Great Masticator." Times of India,July 19, 2013. Accessed June 10, 2017. https://timesofindia.indiatimes.com/life-style/health-fitness/diet/Why-chew-food-thoroughly/articleshow/11912234.cms

https://www.usatoday.com/story/news/nation/2013/04/17/health-food-portion-control/2091865/.

Goff, Ronnie. "Passeggiata to Prevent Diabetes." Awaken Health Fitness. Last modified January 1, 2016. Accessed June 10, 2016. http://awakenhealthfitness.com/passeggiata-prevent-diabetes/

Holla, Anand. "The Great Masticator." Times of India,July 19, 2013. Accessed June 10, 2017. https://timesofindia.indiatimes.com/life-style/health-fitness/diet/Why-chew-food-thoroughly/articleshow/11912234.cms

Kreider, R. B., et al. "A Carbohydrate-restricted Diet During Resistance Training Promotes More Favorable Changes in Body Composition and Markers of Health in Obese Women with and Without Insulin

Resistance." The Physician and Sportsmedicine39, no. 2(May 2011). Accessed July 28, 2017. doi: 10.3810/psm.2011.05.1893.

"MacDonald Talks 300: Rise of a Warrior Challenge, 300 Sequel, Batman vs. Superman Training." Moviehole.com. Accessed July 29, 2017. http://moviehole.net/201473018macdonald-talks-300-rise-of-a-warrior-challenge-300-sequel-batman-vs-superman-training.

Milo, Ron. "How Quickly do Different Cells in the Body Replace Themselves." Cell Biology by the Numbers. Accessed June 11, 2017. http://book.bionumbers.org/how-quickly-do-different-cells-in-the-body-replace-themselves/

Mobbs, Charles, et al. "Treatment of Diabetes and Diabetic Complications with a Ketogenic Diet." *Journal of Child Neurology* 28, no. 8 (August 28, 2013). Accessed July 28, 2017.doi: 10.1177/0883073813487596.

Palmnas, M. S., et al. "Low-Dose Aspartame Consumption Differentially Affects Gut Microbiota-Host Metabolic Interactions in the Diet-Induced Obese Rat." PLOS ONE9, no. 10 (October 2014). Accessed June 10, 2017. doi: 10.1371/journal.pone.0109841.

Rosedale, Ron. "Burn Fat, Not Sugar, to Lose Weight." Mercola. Last modified June 9, 2005. Accessed July 29, 2017. http://articles.mercola.com/sites/articles/archive/2005/06/09/fatburn.aspx

28, no. 8 (August 28, 2013). Accessed July 28, 2017.doi: 10.1177/0883073813487596.

Palmnas, M. S., et al. "Low-Dose Aspartame Consumption Differentially Affects Gut Microbiota-Host Metabolic Interactions in the Diet-Induced Obese Rat." PLOS ONE9, no. 10 (October 2014). Accessed June 10, 2017. doi: 10.1371/journal.pone.0109841.

Rosedale, Ron. "Burn Fat, Not Sugar, to Lose Weight." Mercola. Last modified June 9, 2005. Accessed July 29, 2017. http://articles.mercola.com/sites/articles/archive/2005/06/09/fatburn.aspx

Rubin, Gretchen. The Happiness Project. New York: Harper Paperbacks, 2009.

"Sleep and Health." *Healthy Sleep*. Harvard Medical School. Last modified January 16, 2008. Accessed June 5, 2017. http://healthysleep.med.harvard.edu/need-sleep/whats-in-it-for-you/health.

Suez, J., et al. "Artificial Sweeteners Induce Glucose Intolerance by Altering the Gut Microbiota." Nature 514 (October 2014). Accessed June 10, 2017. doi:10.1038/nature13793 2014.

Weaver, Libby. "The Science and Impact of Rushing." *DrLibby.* Accessed July 6, 2017. https://www.drlibby.com/science-impact-rushing/.

Weil, Andrew. "Breathing Exercises: 4-7-8:Breath." *DrWeilvideo,* 3:18. Accessed July 6, 2017. https://www.drweil.com/videos-features/videos/breathing-exercises-4-7-8-breath/.

Whiteman, Honor. "The Benefit of Chewing Your Food More." Medical News Today, July 19, 2013. Accessed June 10, 2017. https://www.medicalnewstoday.com/articles/263541.php.

Wood, Tommy. "Sit Less and Prioritize Movement for Long-Term Fitness." Breaking Muscle. Accessed July 17, 2017. http://breakingmuscle.com/fitness/sit-less-and-prioritize-movement-for-long-term-fitness.

Whiteman, Honor. "The Benefit of Chewing Your Food More." *Medical News Today*, July 19, 2013. Accessed June 10, 2017. https://www.medicalnewstoday.com/articles/263541.php.

Wood, Tommy. "Sit Less and Prioritize Movement for Long-Term Fitness." *Breaking Muscle*. Accessed July 17, 2017. http://breakingmuscle.com/fitness/sit-less-and-prioritize-movement-for-long-term-fitness.

The Institute for Integrative Nutrition® teaches the term "bio-individuality," which is the concept that no one diet or lifestyle works for everyone. Each person's nutritional needs are individual, and based on a number of varying factors such as lifestyle, occupation, climate, age, gender, culture, and religion. Lifestyle needs are individual as well; what works for one person may not work for another with regard to relationships, exercise, career, spirituality, and physical activity. Additionally, people's needs change over time, so it is important to check in with yourself as you evolve.

www.ingramcontent.com/pod-product-compliance
Lightning Source LLC
Chambersburg PA
CBHW060804270326
41927CB00002B/41